Pocket Examiner in
Obstetrics and Gynaecology

Pocket Examiner
in
Obstetrics and Gynaecology

Peter Bowen-Simpkins
David Pugh

Churchill Livingstone

EDINBURGH LONDON MELBOURNE AND NEW YORK 1987

CHURCHILL LIVINGSTONE
Medical Division of Longman Group UK Limited

Distributed in the United States of America by
Churchill Livingstone Inc., 1560 Broadway, New York,
N.Y. 10036, and by associated companies, branches
and representatives throughout the world.

First published 1983 (Pitman Publishing Ltd)
    Reprinted 1984, 1985
    Reprinted 1987 (Churchill Livingstone)

ISBN   0-443-03844-9

British Library Cataloguing in Publication Data
Bowen-Simpkins, Peter
    Pocket examiner in obstetrics and gynaecology.
    1. Gynecology—Examinations, questions, answers etc.
    2. Obstetrics—Examinations, questions, answers etc.
    I. Title   II. Pugh, David
    618'.076   RC111

Library of Congress Cataloging in Publication Data
Bowen-Simpkins, Peter
    Pocket examiner in obstetrics and gynaecology.
    Bibliography: p.
    1. Obstetrics—Handbooks, manuals, etc.
    2. Gynecology—Handbooks, manuals, etc.   I. Pugh,
    David (David Robert)   II. Title.   [DNLM: 1.
    Gynecology—Examination questions.
    2. Obstetrics—Examination questions. WQ 18 B786p]
    RG531.B68   1983   618'.076   82–9106
                        AACR2

Printed in Great Britain at The Bath Press, Avon

Contents

Preface   vii

Acknowledgements   ix

1   Key to References and Further Reading   1

2   **Questions**   **3**
    Obstetrics   3–36
    A   Basis of ante natal care   3
    B   Assessment of fetal well-being   7
    C   Ante natal disorders of
        pregnancy   11
    D   Normal labour   22
    E   Disorders of labour   28
    F   The puerperium   33
    G   Maternal and perinatal mortality
        statistics   34
    H   The neonate   35

    Gynaecology   36–54
    A   Anatomy of the female reproductive
        organs   36
    B   Physiology of menstruation   37
    C   Disorders associated with the
        menstrual cycle   37
    D   Intersex   39
    E   Amenorrhoea, virilism and
        hirsutism   39
    F   Abortion, ectopic pregnancy and
        trophoblastic disease   40
    G   Diseases of the vulva   42
    H   Diseases of the vagina   43
    I   Diseases of the cervix   44
    J   Diseases of the uterus   46
    K   Diseases of the fallopian tubes   47
    L   Diseases of the ovaries   48
    M   Endometriosis   49
    N   Uterine displacements, prolapse and
        associated urinary problems   49
    O   The climacteric and menopause   50
    P   Fertility control   51

3 **Answers** 55
    Obstetrics 55–170
      A Basis of ante natal care 55
      B Assessment of fetal well-being 69
      C Ante natal disorders of pregnancy 82
      D Normal labour 117
      E Disorders of labour 139
      F The puerperium 157
      G Maternal and perinatal mortality statistics 163
      H The neonate 165

    Gynaecology 170–243
      A Anatomy of the female reproductive organs 170
      B Physiology of menstruation 173
      C Disorders associated with the menstrual cycle 175
      D Intersex 180
      E Amenorrhoea, virilism and hirsutism 182
      F Abortion, ectopic pregnancy and trophoblastic disease 186
      G Diseases of the vulva 195
      H Diseases of the vagina 199
      I Diseases of the cervix 201
      J Diseases of the uterus 209
      K Diseases of the fallopian tubes 214
      L Diseases of the ovaries 218
      M Endometriosis 222
      N Uterine displacements, prolapse and associated urinary problems 226
      O The climacteric and menopause 230
      P Fertility control 233

Preface

This pocket book is primarily aimed at the final year medical student who is revising for his or her written and oral examination in obstetrics and gynaecology. Like the others in this series, it is not intended to replace the standard textbooks available in the subject. It is hoped that the questions posed are those that a student might expect to be asked in his examination; the answers are complete in themselves but references to standard texts are given, and where depth may have been sacrificed for the sake of brevity, the reader will need to turn to these books for further reading.

One problem that is inherent in writing a book of this nature is a tendency to provide answers which read as lists. We tried to avoid this as far as possible but in certain instances it has been impossible by the very nature of the question posed.

In any clinical field, change is always occurring. Some of the answers we have given are based on latest research and, to a lesser degree, personal experience, and therefore may not reflect exactly the opinions expressed in the larger texts to which we refer. In a clinical subject like obstetrics it is almost impossible to give a consensus of opinion in certain areas but we hope that by diversifying his or her reading the student may arrive at a balanced view. It is with these aims in mind that we trust that this book will offer some stimulation as well as pure revision.

PB-S
DP

Acknowledgements

We would like to offer our thanks to our wives for their encouragement in this joint venture and to Mrs Christine Watson and Mrs Delina Dawson for their thankless task of having to decipher our hand writing and for typing and retyping the manuscript. They have done this with evident pleasure and enthusiasm, even when confronted with an enormous load at short notice, and we are most grateful.

It has been most satisfying to work with the publishers, who have shown great forbearance and offered invaluable help.

1
Key to references and further reading

A   *Williams Obstetrics*, Pritchard, J. A. and Mac-
     Donald, P. C., 16th edn. (Appleton Century
     Crofts, New York, 1980)

B   *Obstetrics and the Newborn*, Beischer , N. A. and
     Mackay,   E.   V.,   British   edn.   (Saunders,
     Eastbourne, 1978)

C   *Integrated Obstetrics and Gynaecology for Postgradu-
     ates*, Dewhurst, Sir John, 3rd edn. (Blackwell
     Scientific Publications, Oxford, 1981)

D   *Fundamentals   of   Obstetrics   and   Gynaecology*,
     Llewellyn Jones, Derek, 3rd edn. Vol. I *Obstetrics*.
     (Faber and Faber Ltd, London, 1982)

E   *Fundamentals   of   Obstetrics   and   Gynaecology*,
     Llewellyn Jones, Derek, Vol. II *Gynaecology*.
     (Faber and Faber Ltd, London, 1982)

F   *Obstetrics by Ten Teachers*, Clayton, Sir Stanley G.,
     Lewis, T. L. T., Pinker, G. D., 13th edn. (Edward
     Arnold, London, 1980)

G   *Gynaecology by Ten Teachers*, Clayton, Sir Stanley
     G., Lewis T. L. T., Pinker, G. D., 13th edn.
     (Edward Arnold, London, 1980)

H   *Novak's Textbook of Gynaecology*, Jones, Howard W.
     and   Jones,   Georgeanna   Seegar,   10th   edn.
     (Williams and Wilkins, Baltimore/London, 1981)

I   *Practical Obstetrical Problems*, Donald, I., 5th edn.
     (Lloyd-Luke, London, 1979)

J   *Principles of Gynaecology*, Jeffcoate, Sir Norman,
     4th edn. (Butterworths, London/Boston, 1975)

2
Questions

OBSTETRICS

A   Basis of ante natal care

Physiology of reproduction

1   Define conception.

2   What is the meaning of the terms haploid and diploid chromosome content?

3   How is the haploid number of chromosomes achieved?

4   What do you understand by the term decidua?

5   What aids transport of the ovum to the fallopian tube?

6   Where does fertilisation normally take place?

7   Describe the development of the fertilised ovum prior to implantation.

8   At what stage of development does the fertilised egg enter the uterine cavity?

9   Following implantation what is the next stage in trophoblast differentiation?

10   What happens to the inner cell mass?

11   What structures are developed from each layer of the inner cell mass?

12   At what stage does the embryo become a fetus?

13   What is the early function of the cyto-trophoblast?

14   What are the functions of the placenta?

15   How does transport of substances through the placenta take place?

Maternal physiology

16 What is the maximal weight increase that can be expected in an uncomplicated pregnancy?

17 What changes occur in plasma volume in pregnancy?

18 What happens to cardiac output in pregnancy?

19 How is the increased cardiac output of pregnancy maintained?

20 What is the cause of supine hypotension?

21 There is an increase in red cell mass in pregnancy. What is responsible for this increase?

22 What changes occur in blood coagulation during pregnancy?

23 What changes in renal function occur in pregnancy?

24 What is the effect of pregnancy on the respiratory system?

25 What changes may occur in the alimentary tract during pregnancy?

Anatomy

26 What types of pelvis are commonly encountered in obstetrics and what is the variation in the shape of the pelvic brim?

27 How does an android pelvis differ from a gynaecoid pelvis?

28 What is the pelvic brim?

29 What do you understand by the term obstetric conjugate?

30 What do you understand by the term vertex?

31 What percentage of babies are born by the vertex?

32 What is the biparietal diameter of the fetal skull?

33 What is the pelvic floor comprised of?

Diagnosis of pregnancy

34 What are the early symptoms of pregnancy?

35 What are the early signs of pregnancy?

36 What is the pigmentation of facial skin seen in pregnancy known as?

37 What are pregnancy tests dependent upon?

38 When does the pregnancy test become negative?

39 When are fetal movements usually first felt?

40 When can fetal parts be first palpated?

Ante natal care

41 What are the aims of ante natal care?

42 What is the difference between a primiparous patient and a primigravid patient?

43 When should the first ante natal visit be made to the obstetrician?

44 How often should a patient be seen ante natally?

45 What information should be obtained from the history taken at the first ante natal visit?

46 What would routine examination at the first ante natal visit entail?

47 What information can be gained from a vaginal examination and bimanual examination at the first ante natal visit?

48 Are there occasions when such an examination should be omitted?

49 What are the routine blood tests carried out at the first visit to an ante natal clinic?

50 What routine observations are made at each ante natal visit which might enable detection of the fetus at risk?

51 What are the likely causes of proteinuria?

52 What would you regard as an abnormal blood pressure recording in pregnancy?

53 What are the dangers of excessive weight gain in pregnancy?

54 What is the significance of poor weight gain in pregnancy?

55 What is the significance of bleeding in the mid trimester of pregnancy?

56 What is the effect of smoking on pregnancy?

57 Should intercourse be forbidden at any stage of pregnancy?

58 What is the cause of heartburn in pregnancy?

59 How can heartburn be treated in pregnancy?

60 What are the causes of vaginal discharge in pregnancy?

61 How can a woman with inverted nipples, who wishes to breastfeed, be helped in pregnancy?

62 What is the cause of varicose veins in pregnancy?

63 What information can be obtained from abdominal palpation in the latter half of pregnancy?

64 What is Pawlik's grip (palpation)?

65 What does engagement mean?

66 What are the causes for non-engagement of the fetal head at term?

67 Is there any value in obtaining a lateral X-ray of

the pelvis when the fetus presents by the head and you suspect cephalopelvic disproportion on a primigravid patient?

Uterine displacements and anomalies

68   You perform a bimanual vaginal examination on a patient who is 8 weeks pregnant. She has a mobile ovarian cyst about 5 cm in diameter to the right of the uterus. What is your management?

69   How would you deal with an ovarian cyst detected after the 29th week of pregnancy?

70   What is the likely diagnosis in a patient with acute retention of urine in the early part of the second trimester of pregnancy?

71   What are the possible effects of fibroids (myomata) on pregnancy?

72   What are the possible effects of fibroids (myomata) on labour?

73   What are the common congenital anomalies of the female genital tract?

74   Do abnormalities of the uterus influence the outcome of pregnancy?

B   Assessment of fetal well-being

Amniocentesis, prenatal diagnosis and genetics

75   What means are there for screening for neural tube defects?

76   What are the limitations of α-fetoprotein (AFP) measurements in maternal serum?

77   What other conditions give rise to raised serum AFP levels?

78   What other potential obstetric problem may be highlighted by a raised serum AFP?

79　In what way is it thought that neural tube defects can be prevented?

80　What are the indications for mid trimester amniocentesis?

81　At what stage in the second trimester is amniocentesis usually first performed?

82　What information may be obtained from amniotic fluid aspirated in the second and third trimesters of pregnancy?

83　What are the dangers of amniocentesis?

84　What other disorders may be identified by amniocentesis?

85　What is the most common chromosomal abnormality seen at birth?

86　What influence does maternal age have on the risk of Down's syndrome occurring?

87　If both parents carry a recessive gene, what is the incidence of affected children?

88　If a female is carrying a sex-linked abnormal gene, how will the children be affected?

89　What is non-disjunction?

90　What is translocation?

91　Give examples of a dominantly inherited genetic disorder.

92　Give some examples of X-linked recessive disorders.

Assessment of gestational age

93　How do you calculate the estimated date of delivery (EDD)?

94　What circumstances can lead to an erroneous calculation of the EDD?

95　If you suspect a woman has 'wrong dates' how

would you estimate the duration of the pregnancy?

96   What are the causes of a patient being 'large-for-dates' in the second trimester?

97   What tests are available for assessment of fetal maturity in the third trimester?

98   There is a sudden increase in the lecithin sphyngomyelin ratio (LSR) at 28 weeks' gestation which subsequently falls and does not rise again until 34 weeks. Why does this occur?

99   Under what circumstances can a fetus with an amniotic LSR of 2:1 or greater, develop respiratory distress syndrome?

100   What are the radiological signs of fetal death?

Placental insufficiency

101   The term primary and secondary placental dysfunction is sometimes used. What does this mean?

102   What are the common causes of placental dysfunction in pregnancy?

103   What groups of patients require close monitoring to detect intrauterine growth retardation (IUGR)?

104   What clinical signs can help us identify growth retardation in apparently normal pregnancies?

105   What effect does IUGR have on babies' development?

106   How can the increased mortality and morbidity of the growth retarded fetus be reduced?

Ante partum tests

107   What methods of assessing fetal well-being are currently available?

108 Is there any significance in a reduction in maternally observed fetal movements after the 32nd week of pregnancy?

109 What are the uses of ultrasound scanning in the second trimester of pregnancy?

110 What are the important uses of ultrasound in the third trimester?

111 Are there any other measurements which might be even more successful at diagnosing intra-uterine growth retardation (IUGR)?

112 Of what use is human placental lactogen (HPL) estimation in monitoring fetal well-being?

113 What are the advantages and disadvantages of oestriol estimations in the third trimester?

114 What factors can affect total oestrogen concentrations?

115 The value of assessment of fetal well-being based on hormone assays has been questioned. Why should this be so?

116 What is a cardiotocograph?

117 What do you understand by the term ante natal stress test?

118 What are the advantages of ante natal un-stressed cardiotocography?

119 What criteria should be satisfied for an ante natal cardiotocograph (CTG) to be judged normal?

120 In what way may fetal breathing patterns indicate fetal jeopardy?

Intrapartum monitoring

121 What methods are available for monitoring uterine contractions?

122 What do you understand by fetal distress in labour?

123 What methods are available for monitoring fetal heart rate (FHR)?

124 What do you accept as a normal fetal heart rate pattern in labour?

125 What is beat-to-beat variation?

126 What abnormalities of the FHR pattern may be described?

127 How do you define baseline bradycardia?

128 How do you define baseline tachycardia?

129 What is a type 1 dip?

130 What is a type 2 dip?

131 What are variable decelerations?

132 What are the major causes of fetal hypoxia in labour?

133 Fetal heart rate abnormalities may suggest fetal hypoxia. How may this be confirmed?

134 Why should pH estimation reflect hypoxia?

135 Describe the technique of fetal blood sampling (FBS).

136 How may the results of FBS be interpreted?

137 In what way may the fetus be compromised during uterine contractions?

C Ante natal disorders of pregnancy

Systemic diseases—cardiac

138 What is the main aim of ante natal management of patients with heart disease?

139 A systolic murmur is heard at routine booking clinic examination. What course of action should be taken?

140 What are the four classes of cardiac function in heart disease?

141 What grounds are there for termination of pregnancy in a patient with heart disease?

142 What are the main causes of heart disease in pregnancy?

143 What effect will pregnancy have on patients with heart disease?

144 Does heart disease have any effect on pregnancy?

145 What is the indication for cardiac surgery in pregnancy?

146 What precautions should be taken with a cardiac patient in labour?

147 What other measures should be taken in the first stage of labour in the cardiac patient?

148 What analgesia would you advise for the first stage of labour in a patient with cardiac disease?

149 How would you conduct the second stage of labour in a patient with cardiac disease?

150 How should the third stage of labour be managed in the cardiac patient?

151 What are the indications for anticoagulants in a patient with heart disease?

152 Is there a place for induction of labour in patients with cardiac disease?

153 Summarise how you would manage the labour of a patient with mild mitral stenosis (grades I and II)

Systemic diseases—anaemia

154 What happens to erythropoiesis in pregnancy?

155 What is the lowest acceptable value of haemoglobin in late pregnancy?

156 What are the benefits of prophylactic iron therapy during pregnancy?

157 What do you regard as satisfactory prophylactic treatment of anaemia in pregnancy?

158 What are the two most common anaemias of pregnancy?

159 What are the common causes of iron deficiency anaemia in pregnancy?

160 What investigations would you carry out on a patient with haemoglobin below 10·5 g per 100 ml?

161 What effects does iron deficiency anaemia have on pregnancy?

162 How do you treat iron deficiency anaemia in pregnancy?

163 How would you treat a patient who is 34 weeks pregnant and has a haemoglobin of 9·8 g/100 ml due to iron deficiency?

164 How would you treat severe anaemia after 36 weeks' gestation?

165 What factors may cause megaloblastic anaemia in pregnancy?

166 How may folic acid deficiency or megaloblastic anaemia be diagnosed?

167 Why is folic acid needed in the diet?

168 What effects may folic acid deficiency have on pregnancy?

169 What is sickle cell disease?

170 What are the dangers of sickle cell anaemia in pregnancy?

171 How should a patient with sickle cell disease be managed?

172 How would you treat the anaemia of a patient suffering from thalassaemia?

173 What effect does idiopathic thrombocytopenic purpura have on pregnancy?

174 What advice would you give to a woman with Hodgkin's disease regarding pregnancy?

Systemic diseases—diabetes

175 What happens to carbohydrate metabolism in pregnancies?

176 What is the incidence of diabetes mellitus in women of childbearing age?

177 How does the fetus respond to raised levels of glucose in the maternal circulation?

178 How can one screen for diabetes in pregnancy?

179 How would you manage a pregnant patient who presents for the first time with glycosuria?

180 Under what circumstances would you perform a glucose tolerance test (GTT) in pregnancy?

181 How would you perform a GTT?

182 What are your criteria for an abnormal GTT?

183 Why do many women who exhibit glycosuria in pregnancy have a normal GTT?

184 What relevance is a first line family history of diabetes?

185 What is the significance to the mother of delivering a baby larger than 4·5 kg?

186 Give a classification of diabetes in pregnancy.

187 What are the effects of diabetes on a pregnancy?

188 What are the effects of pregnancy on diabetes?

189 How are clinical diabetics managed ante natally?

190 What is the place of oral hypoglycaemic agents in pregnancy?

191 How is labour managed in the insulin-dependent diabetic?

192 What is the effect of maternal diabetes mellitus on the baby at birth?

Systemic diseases—urinary tract

193 Why are urinary tract infections more common in pregnancy?

194 What is the incidence of bacteriuria in pregnancy?

195 How would you manage a patient with asymptomatic bacteriuria?

196 Can ureteric colic occur in pregnancy?

197 What are the causes of haematuria in pregnancy and labour?

198 What is the nephrotic syndrome and what is the likely outcome of pregnancy in an affected patient?

Systemic diseases—jaundice

199 What are the causes of jaundice in pregnancy?

200 How may acute fatty necrosis of the liver in pregnancy present?

201 How may intrahepatic cholestatic jaundice present?

202 What effect does pregnancy have on pre-existing liver disease?

203 What drugs may cause jaundice in pregnancy?

204 What happens to liver function in pregnancy?

Systemic diseases—thyroid and adrenal

205 What is the most useful investigation in a case of suspected thyroid disease?

206 What specific investigations should be carried out on cord blood of infants born to mothers receiving antithyroid therapy?

207 Women who have had thyrotoxicosis in the past but who are no longer hyperthyroid can give birth to infants with neonatal thyrotoxicosis. Why?

208 How often is a simple colloid goitre encountered in pregnancy?

209 How should a patient with a solitary nodular thyroid enlargement be managed in pregnancy?

210 A patient develops a diffuse hard irregular goitre during pregnancy and is euthyroid. What might you suspect?

211 What are the effects of hypothyroidism in pregnancy?

212 How is a patient with moderate thyrotoxicosis managed in pregnancy?

213 What problems are associated with Addison's disease and pregnancy?

214 What are the problems of steroid therapy in pregnancy?

215 What is the effect of pregnancy on a phaeo-chromocytoma?

Systemic diseases—respiratory

216 How may pulmonary tuberculosis (TB) be diag-nosed in pregnancy?

217 What effects does pregnancy have on TB?

218 How would you manage a case of TB in pregnancy?

219 A patient presents with a history of recurrent spontaneous pneumothorax. How would you manage her in labour?

220 What problems may pneumonia present in pregnancy?

221 What is the effect of pregnancy on bronchial asthma?

Systemic diseases—sexually transmitted diseases

222 What are the effects of syphilis on a pregnancy?

223 How would you treat syphilis in pregnancy?

224 How may gonorrhoea be detected in pregnancy?

225 What is the treatment for gonorrhoea?

226 What is gonoccocal ophthalmia?

227 How would you treat *Trichomonas vaginalis* infection in pregnancy?

Systemic diseases—abdominal pain

228 To what painful abdominal conditions does pregnancy predispose?

229 What are the causes of pain due to pregnancy in each of the three trimesters?

230 What co-incidental causes of abdominal pain must be considered in pregnancy?

231 How would you differentiate between appendicitis and a renal tract infection in pregnancy?

232 What are the presenting signs and symptoms of red degeneration of a fibroid in pregnancy?

Systemic diseases—viral

233 What is the incidence of major congenital malformations if a patient develops rubella in the first trimester?

234 What are the common defects found in a fetus infected by rubella between the 5th and 14th weeks of pregnancy?

235 How would you manage a patient who has been in contact with rubella (German measles) in the 7th week of her pregnancy?

236 What are the affects of a cytomegalovirus infection (CMV) in pregnancy?

237 What effect does herpes virus have on pregnancy?

238 What effect do the myxoviruses have on pregnancy (mumps, measles and influenza)?

Systemic diseases—neurological

239 What is the effect of pregnancy on epilepsy?

240 What effect does pregnancy have on myasthenia gravis?

241 How would you manage and deliver a patient with myasthenia gravis in pregnancy?

242 What effect does pregnancy have on multiple sclerosis?

243 How may cerebral tumours present in pregnancy?

244 Why are peripheral nerve disorders more common in pregnancy?

Systemic diseases—bowel, skin, psychiatric, drug administration

245 What complications may arise during pregnancy in the patient with ulcerative colitis?

246 How may pregnancy be affected in Crohn's disease?

247 What psychiatric disorders may occur in pregnancy?

248 How may pregnancy psychosis be recognised in the early stages?

249 What common skin rashes are seen in pregnancy?

250 What antibiotics can be safely administered to a pregnant patient?

251 What anticoagulants can be used in pregnancy?

Diseases of pregnancy—hypertension

252 What do you understand by the term pre-eclampsia?

253 What level of hypertension is necessary for a diagnosis to be made?

254 What physiological changes occur in hypertensive disease of pregnancy?

255 What is the aetiology of the disease?

256 What are the other causes of hypertension in pregnancy?

257 What common factors are often associated with the development of hypertensive disease of pregnancy?

258 Clinical examination of the pregnant hypertensive woman should include what features?

259 What laboratory investigations would you carry out in hypertensive pregnancies?

260 What is the medical treatment of hypertensive disease of pregnancy?

261 Under what circumstances should delivery be contemplated in patients with hypertensive disease?

262 A patient has a blood pressure of 140/90 mmHg, and moderate oedema of the ankles at 39 weeks' gestation. What is the management of this patient?

263 How may severe hypertension be controlled in labour?

264 What are the signs of impending eclampsia?

265 How would you manage a pregnant patient with eclampsia?

266 What drugs are commonly used to control eclamptic fits?

Diseases of pregnancy—rhesus disease

267 What is the rhesus factor?

268 How does rhesus isoimmunisation occur?

269 What are the effects of rhesus isoimmunisation on the fetus?

270 How do ABO antibodies differ from rhesus antibodies?

271 Why is rhesus isoimmunisation less common when mother and fetus have differing ABO grouping?

272 Can a rhesus-negative fetus have a rhesus-positive father?

273 What is the routine testing for rhesus antibodies in rhesus-negative women?

274 If a woman has an antibody titre of 1 in 8 or more by the Coombs indirect method (for incomplete antibodies), how is the patient managed?

275 What investigations are carried out at birth, both of mother and the infant?

276 How is rhesus isoimmunisation prevented?

Diseases of pregnancy—hyperemesis gravidarum

277 What is hyperemesis gravidarum?

278 What are the sequelae of hyperemesis gravidarum?

279 How would you treat a case of severe vomiting in pregnancy (hyperemesis gravidarum)?

280 What famous literary figure died from hyper-emesis gravidarum?

Bleeding in pregnancy

281 What is an ante partum haemorrhage?

282 What are the causes of ante partum haemor-rhage?

283 What is placental abruption (abruptio placen-tae)?

284 What aetiological factors are associated with placental abruption?

285 What forms of accidental haemorrhage are there?

286 What is the management of mild degrees of placental abruption, once the diagnosis has been made?

287 How would you manage a case of severe placen-tal abruption?

288 What is a placenta praevia and what types do you know?

289 What is the typical presentation of a patient with placenta praevia?

290 What techniques are available for diagnosing placenta praevia?

291 What is the mangement of mild vaginal bleeding in the third trimester?

292 What is the management of a patient diagnosed as having placenta praevia in the 32nd week of her pregnancy?

293 A patient, who is 38 weeks pregnant, presents with an appreciable painless vaginal haemor-rhage. The fetal head is not engaged and no ultrasonic examination has been made in an otherwise completely normal pregnancy. How would you manage her?

294 What other placental causes of ante partum haemorrhage do you know?

295 What is a vasa praevia?

296 If vaginal bleeding is encountered during labour, how might you determine whether it is fetal or maternal blood?

Liquor amnii

297 What are the functions of the amniotic fluid?

298 What is the approximate volume of liquor at 20 weeks, 36 weeks and term?

299 What is polyhydramnios?

300 What are the common causes of polyhydramnios?

301 How would you manage a patient who develops polyhydramnios in the third trimester?

302 What is the meaning of the term oligohydramnios and what is its significance?

D Normal labour

Physiology

303 What maternal physiological changes occur in labour?

304 What physiological alterations may occur to the fetus during labour?

305 What is the arrangement of muscle fibres in the uterus?

306 What are Braxton Hicks contractions?

307 What factors may initiate labour?

308 From where do the contractions originate in labour?

309 What is the effect of a coordinate uterine contraction?

310 What is the pattern of uterine contractility in pregnancy?

311 What is the meaning of effacement of the cervix?

312 What is the lower segment of the uterus?

313 What is Bandl's ring?

314 What happens to the uterus and lower segment in labour?

315 What causes the pain of uterine contractions?

316 What is the operculum?

317 What is the normal intrauterine resting pressure during pregnancy and labour?

Pain relief

318 What is psychoprophylaxis?

319 What narcotic drugs are commonly used in labour?

320 What are the advantages of narcotic drugs in labour?

321 What is the major side effect of narcotic drugs that are used in labour?

322 What are the main inhalational analgesics available?

323 What is epidural analgesia?

324 What are the major complications of epidural anaesthesia?

325 How would you treat a hypotensive episode occurring immediately after epidural administration?

326 What are the main contraindications to epidural anaesthesia?

327 What are the major complications of general anaesthesia in labour?

328 What is Mendelson's syndrome?

329 What precautions are taken in labour to avoid Mendelson's syndrome?

330 What analgesia may be provided for forceps deliveries?

331 How would you perform a pudendal block?

Diagnosis and first stage

332 What are the three stages of labour?

333 How do you define normal labour?

334 How may labour be recognised?

335 How would you recognise progressive cervical dilatation?

336 Once labour is diagnosed what observations should be undertaken?

337 What important points are assessed at vaginal examination?

338 What is meant by station of the presenting part?

339 How may descent of the fetal head be estimated?

340 What is the significance of the character of the liquor during labour?

341 What is a partogram?

342 What are the two phases commonly described in the first stage of labour?

343 What is the latent phase of labour?

344 How does one determine when the active phase of labour is reached?

345 What is the most common position of the fetal head at the start of labour?

346 What diameter of the fetal skull is presented when the head is flexed?

347 What is asynclitism?

348 What is a caput succedaneum?

349 What is moulding?

Second stage of labour

350 What are the objectives of management of the second stage of labour?

351 What are the external signs of full dilatation of the cervix?

352 What is the average duration of the second stage of labour?

353 How should the patient be managed in the second stage of labour?

354 What positions may be adopted by the patient for delivery?

355 What are the movements that the fetus under-goes to negotiate the birth canal when the head is presenting and is fully flexed?

356 What is crowning?

357 What is meant by restitution?

358 What procedure should be adopted following the birth of the head?

359 After delivery of the head it is noted that the umbilical cord is around the baby's neck (nuchal entanglement), how would you manage such a case?

Third stage of labour

360 What are the mechanisms of placental delivery?

361 In what way may the third stage of labour be managed?

362 What does the physiological management entail?

363 What are the signs that the placenta has separated from the uterus?

364 What are the advantages of physiological management of the third stage of labour?

365 How is the third stage managed actively?

366 What is the Brandt–Andrews technique?

367 What are the advantages of actively managing the third stage of labour?

368 Why is inspection of the placenta important?

369 What is the average weight of the placenta at term?

370 Following delivery, why is cord blood taken when the mother is rhesus negative?

371 Why should the umbilical cord be inspected?

372 What is a velamentous insertion?

373 What is a battledore placenta?

374 What is a circumvallate placenta?

375 What is a succenturiate lobe?

Obstetric operations—induction of labour

376 What methods of induction of labour are available?

377 What are the hindwaters and forewaters?

378 How is forewater amniotomy (rupture of the membranes) performed?

379 What problems may be encountered with oxytocic administration?

380 How may prostaglandins be administered to induce labour?

381 What are the two major reasons for inducing labour?

382 What are the more common indications for induction of labour?

383 What are the complications of induction of labour?

384 What are the contraindications to induction of labour?

Obstetric operations—episiotomy

385 What does the word episiotomy mean?

386 What are the objectives of an episiotomy?

387 What are the advantages of an episiotomy?

388 What types of episiotomy are there?

389 What are the advantages and disadvantages of the mediolateral or J-shaped episiotomy?

390 What are the advantages and disadvantages of the median episiotomy?

391 What tissues are normally cut when a mediolateral episiotomy is performed?

392 What is a third degree tear?

393 What is the treatment of a third degree tear?

Obstetric operations—instrumental delivery

394 What are the main features of obstetric forceps?

395 What are the indications for forceps delivery?

396 What conditions must be present before forceps delivery is attempted?

397 What complications can arise from forceps delivery?

398 As well as assessing the vaginal findings prior to forceps delivery, it is important to perform one other examination to prevent difficulties arising. What is this examination?

399 What is the ventouse?

400 What are the uses of the ventouse?

Obstetric operations—caesarean section

401 What are the major indications for emergency caesarean section?

402 What are the main maternal complications of caesarean sections?

403 How would you manage the patient with a previous lower segment caesarean section in subsequent pregnancies?

404 What are the signs of impending uterine scar rupture in labour?

405 What are the two types of caesarean section encountered and how do they differ?

406 What are the main indications for classical caesarean section?

Obstetric operations—internal podalic version

407 What do you understand by the term internal podalic version?

408 Under what circumstances may internal podalic version be undertaken?

E   Disorders of labour

Dystocia, augmentation and premature labour

409 What is augmentation of labour?

410 What are the advantages of augmentation of labour?

411 Which group of patients most frequently present with abnormal labour patterns?

412 What is incoordinate hypertonic uterine inertia?

413 What is understood by the term hypotonic uterine inertia and how may inertia be classified?

414 How may the conditions of uterine hypotonia be overcome?

415 How can the condition of incoordinate hypertonic uterine inertia be overcome?

416 How do you define premature labour?

417 What are the main causes of premature labour that progresses to delivery?

418 What preventive measures can be taken in a woman whose uterus is contracting regularly at 34 weeks and you believe to be in labour?

Malpresentations and malpositions

419 The perinatal mortality rate is increased with malpresentations. Why should this be so?

420 What maternal risks are there with malpresentations?

421 What is the commonest malpresentation in labour?

422 What factors are mainly responsible for the occipitoposterior presentation?

423 How might an occipitoposterior position be diagnosed?

424 What is the character of the labour in occipitoposterior presentations?

425 Why should labour in occipitoposterior presentations be more prolonged and painful?

426 What is the usual outcome of labour with the occipitoposterior positions?

427 If the occipitoposterior position persists to full dilatation, what methods of delivery can be contemplated?

428 How would you manage a deep transverse arrest of the occiput?

429 What is the incidence of multiple pregnancy?

430 How can you distinguish a monozygotic (uniovular) pregnancy from a dizygotic (binovular) pregnancy at birth?

431 Do both infants present by the head in the majority of twin pregnancies?

432 What is a fetus papyraceus?

433 How is a diagnosis of multiple pregnancy made clinically?

434 What other methods are available for the diagnosis of twins?

435 What problems occur more frequently in multiple pregnancies?

436 How can premature onset of labour be prevented in multiple pregnancy?

437 What staff must be present at the delivery of twins?

438 How should the second stage of a twin delivery be conducted?

439 What are the dangers to the second twin following delivery of the first?

440 If the second twin was found to be lying in a transverse position after delivery of the first, what would you do?

441 What is the incidence of breech presentation?

442 What is the aetiology of breech presentation?

443 How do you diagnose a breech presentation?

444 What types of breech presentations are there?

445 What is the management of the breech presentation ante natally?

446 How would you conduct a vaginal breech delivery?

447 How long a delay should there be between delivery of the trunk and arms and delivery of the head?

448 What is the Mauriceau–Smellie–Veit manoeuvre?

449 What are the causes of death associated with breech delivery?

450 What is the major complication when a patient presents in labour with a footling breech?

451 What other malpresentations, other than breech and twins, may be encountered in labour?

452 What is the aetiology of face and brow presentation?

453 What is the normal course of labour in face presentation?

454 What is the normal course of labour in brow presentation?

455 What is the incidence of oblique and transverse lie?

456 What aetiological factors predispose towards oblique and transverse lies?

457 How is this condition managed ante natally?

458 What are the hazards of a transverse lie in labour?

459 How would you manage a transverse lie in labour?

460 Are there any instances when vaginal delivery of a transverse lie may be possible?

461 What is a compound presentation?

Obstetric emergencies—cord prolapse

462   What factors predispose to cord prolapse?

463   What immediate action would you take if you made a diagnosis of cord prolapse?

464   What other measures are necessary if cord prolapse is discovered?

465   What is the prognosis for the baby following cord prolapse?

Post partum haemorrhage

466   What is a primary post partum haemorrhage?

467   What are the main causes of primary post partum haemorrhage?

468   What are the causes of uterine atony?

469   How may uterine atony be overcome?

470   How is a patient with retained products of conception managed?

471   If the placenta is retained for 15 minutes after delivery of the child, what measures should be taken?

472   What is placenta accreta and what is the cause?

473   If a patient is bleeding continuously following completion of the third stage, what steps must be taken?

Uterine rupture; impacted shoulders; uterine inversion; defects of coagulation

474   What factors predispose to uterine rupture?

475   What action must be taken if rupture is suspected?

476   What do you understand by the term shoulder dystocia and how would you manage such a problem?

477 Explain the meaning of the term uterine inversion.

478 How might uterine inversion be managed?

479 What are the more common aetiological causes of defects of coagulation in pregnancy?

480 What is an amniotic fluid embolism?

481 What is the pathology of the condition?

F The puerperium

482 How do you define the puerperium?

483 What is meant by involution?

484 What do you understand by the term lochial discharge?

485 What is colostrum?

486 Why can breastfeeding only be established after birth?

487 Would you expect lactation to occur after a spontaneous abortion?

488 What happens to prolactin levels in the puerperium?

489 Why is breast milk the ideal food for the baby?

490 Are there anti-infective agents present in breast milk?

491 Are there any contraindications to breast-feeding?

492 What methods are used for the suppression of lactation?

493 How do you define puerperal infection?

494 How often does puerperal infection occur and what are the usual sites of infection?

495 How would you investigate a patient with puerperal pyrexia?

496 What organisms are commonly responsible for puerperal infection?

497 When does menstruation return in breastfeeding and non-breastfeeding mothers?

498 What degree of contraception does lactation afford the breastfeeding mother?

499 Why is conception less likely during lactation?

500 How are cracked nipples treated?

501 What urinary complications may arise in the puerperium?

502 What aetiological factors are involved in venous thrombosis in pregnancy?

503 What prophylactic measures may be undertaken during pregnancy to prevent thrombosis occurring?

504 What percentage of patients develop venous thrombosis in the puerperium?

505 How do you treat superficial and deep venous thrombosis?

506 What is the object of the post natal examination?

507 A patient presents at her 6-week post natal visit and gives a history of recurrent bright red vaginal loss. What is the differential diagnosis?

G Maternal and perinatal mortality statistics

508 What is the definition of maternal mortality?

509 What are the most common causes of maternal death?

510 There has been a considerable fall in maternal mortality rate over the last 40 years. What factors may account for this?

511 How would you define the perinatal mortality rate (PMR)?

512 What is the PMR in England and Wales at the present time?

513 What are the main causes of perinatal death?

514 What factors may influence the perinatal mortality rate?

H   The neonate

515 What is the average weight and head circumference of a baby at birth?

516 What is an Apgar score?

517 What action should be taken if a baby has a low Apgar score?

518 What measures should be taken if an asphyxiated baby is delivered covered in meconium?

519 How may the gestational age of the infant be assessed following delivery?

520 How do you classify low birth weight babies?

521 What are the clinical differences that can be detected between premature and low birth weight babies?

522 What problems may the low birth weight infant encounter?

523 Define respiratory distress. What are the main causes?

524 What are the general principles in management of a baby with respiratory distress syndrome (hyaline membrane disease HMD)?

525 Oxygen therapy is not without risk. What problems may be caused and how may this be prevented?

526 Jaundice is commonly seen in the newborn baby. Why should this be so?

527 What are some of the main causes of jaundice in the neonate?

528 Under what circumstances does jaundice require investigation or action?

529 What methods are available for reducing serum bilirubin levels?

530 What do you understand by the term kernicterus?

531 What is the significance of IgM antibodies in a baby at birth?

532 Ortolani and Guthrie tests are carried out in the newborn infant. What are these tests seeking to establish?

GYNAECOLOGY

A   Anatomy of the female reproductive organs

533 What structures may be included in the term the vulva?

534 What is the vestibule?

535 What is the perineal body?

536 What are the main relations of the uterus?

537 What are the main supports of the uterus?

538 From where do the ovaries receive their blood supply?

539 Describe the venous drainage of the ovaries.

540 What is the normal sequence of events in normal sexual differentiation?

541 What determines whether the gonad becomes a testis or an ovary?

542 What is the name given to the embryological ducts which temporarily coexist in all embryos?

543 What determines which duct system will develop?

544 What determines external genitalia differentiation?

B Physiology of menstruation

545 What glands are involved in the control of the menstrual cycle?

546 What controls the levels of ovarian oestrogen during the menstrual cycle?

547 What hormonal event immediately precedes ovulation?

548 After ovulation, what are the predominant hormones that the ovary produces and from what cells?

549 Why do FSH levels fall a few days prior to ovulation?

550 What is the action of oestrogen on the uterus?

551 What is the effect of oestrogens on the vagina?

552 What action does progesterone have on the endometrium?

553 What are the main oestrogens found in the circulation?

554 What is the mechanism of menstrual bleeding?

555 What changes occur in vaginal epithelium through the menstrual cycle?

C Disorders associated with the menstrual cycle

556 What is the premenstrual syndrome (PMS)?

557 What are the aetiological factors in PMS?

558 What treatment is available to sufferers?

559 What is idiopathic oedema of women?

560 What is dysmenorrhoea?

561 What characterises spasmodic dysmenorrhoea?

562 What is the treatment of spasmodic dysmenorrhoea?

563 What are the causes of congestive dysmenorrhoea?

564 What is Mittelschmerz?

565 What do you understand by dysfunctional uterine bleeding?

566 Assuming that there is an endocrinological basis to the abnormal bleeding, how may you classify this?

567 What clinical investigations would you undertake before diagnosing dysfunctional uterine bleeding?

568 What forms of treatment are available for dysfunctional bleeding?

569 What forms of hormonal therapy are available for dysfunctional bleeding?

570 What is metropathia haemorrhagica?

571 What are the histological features of the endometrium in metropathia haemorrhagica?

572 What forms of therapy are available for dysfunctional uterine haemorrhage, other than hormonal?

573 What are the causes of postmenopausal bleeding?

574 What investigations must be carried out in cases of postmenopausal bleeding?

575 How would you perform a diagnostic curettage?

576 What are the causes of postcoital bleeding?

D Intersex

577 What four factors govern the sex of a person?

578 In what condition is the gonadal and chromosomal sex male, and the phenotype and gender sex female?

579 What is gonadal dysgenesis?

580 What is adrenogenital syndrome?

581 What is the effect of androgens on the external genitalia of a female fetus?

582 What is Klinefelter's syndrome?

E Amenorrhoea, virilism and hirsutism

583 What is amenorrhoea?

584 What are the most common causes of amenorrhoea?

585 What is an haematocolpos?

586 What are the clinical features of haematocolpos?

587 What gonadal causes of amenorrhoea may occur?

588 What are the endocrine causes of amenorrhoea?

589 When taking a history from a patient with amenorrhoea, what particular points would you enquire about?

590 What laboratory investigations would you undertake?

591 Is there a simple way of assessing oestrogen levels in a patient with primary amenorrhoea?

592 How would you treat a patient with secondary amenorrhoea caused by a hypothalamopituitary disorder (low FSH levels)?

593 What would you look for as a sign of hyper-prolactinaemia in a woman with secondary amenorrhoea?

594 What are the most likely causes of hyperprolactinaemia?

595 How would you treat a patient with hyper-prolactinaemia?

596 What are the characteristics of polycystic ovary syndrome?

597 What organic causes of hirsutism do you know?

598 What laboratory tests would you do in cases of mild or moderate hirsutism with no other evidence of virilism?

599 What is the treatment of hirsutism?

F Abortion, ectopic pregnancy and trophoblastic disease

600 What is abortion?

601 How common is spontaneous abortion?

602 What are the causes of spontaneous abortion?

603 What types of abortion are recognised?

604 What is a threatened abortion and how may it be treated?

605 How does an inevitable abortion differ from an incomplete abortion?

606 What is the treatment of an inevitable or incomplete abortion?

607 What are the major complications of an incomplete abortion?

608 What are the clinical features of a septic abortion?

609 How is a patient with a septic abortion treated?

610 What is a missed abortion?

611 What is the risk of subsequent abortion after one abortion?

612 What is the aetiology of cervical incompetence?

613 When would you suspect that a patient had cervical incompetence?

614 How may cervical incompetence be treated?

615 Prior to the introduction of a cervical suture, what should the patient be told?

616 How may therapeutic termination of pregnancy be carried out in the first trimester of pregnancy?

617 What methods are available for the termination of second trimester pregnancies?

618 What is an ectopic pregnancy?

619 What is the aetiology of the condition?

620 What is the outcome of the pregnancy when it is tubal?

621 What are the clinical features of tubal pregnancy?

622 What other common conditions may cause confusion of diagnosis with ectopic pregnancies?

623 What clinical action would you take in a woman suspected of having an ectopic pregnancy?

624 In a case of ruptured tubal pregnancy, with massive haemorrhage, what should be done?

625 What is the probability of a patient who has had an ectopic pregnancy having a subsequent one?

626 The trophoblast invades the host but that invasion is normally halted. Occasionally this mechanism fails. What is the result?

627 What is the incidence of hydatidiform mole and in what groups of women does it more commonly occur?

628 What is known of the aetiology of trophoblastic disease?

629 Describe the clinical features of a patient with a hydatidiform mole?

630 What is the immediate treatment of a hydatidiform mole?

631 How is a patient with benign trophoblastic disease followed up and what advice should be given with regard to contraception and future pregnancies?

632 What is the aetiology of choriocarcinoma (malignant trophoblastic disease)?

633 Outline the clinical features of choriocarcinoma.

634 Describe briefly the treatment of choriocarcinoma and the survival rates?

635 What is an invasive mole (chorioadenoma destruens)?

G   Diseases of the vulva

636 What is pruritus vulvae?

637 What conditions may lead to pruritus vulvae?

638 In cases where no obvious cause can be found for the pruritus, such as infection, glycosuria, oestrogen depletion etc., what steps should be taken?

639 What is chronic vulval dystrophy?

640 What is the significance of thickened white patches on the vulva?

641 How does preinvasive (intraepithelial) carcinoma of the vulva present?

642 In what age group are you most likely to encounter carcinoma of the vulva?

643 In what way does squamous carcinoma of the vulva present?

644 Are there a number of treatments available for the treatment of the condition?

645 Warts are common in the vulval and perineal region. What conditions are likely to encourage their growth?

646 What treatments are available for condylomata acuminata (warts)?

647 What other benign tumours occur on the vulva?

648 What is a urethral caruncle?

649 What is a Bartholin's cyst?

650 What treatment would you advocate for a Bartholin's cyst?

651 If left untreated, what is the likely outcome of a Bartholin's cyst?

652 What are herpetic ulcers of the vulva?

H   Diseases of the vagina

653 How is the acidity of the vagina maintained?

654 What is leucorrhoea?

655 What are the clinical features of a monilial discharge?

656 What treatment is available for moniliasis?

657 What are the features of a trichomonal vaginal infection?

658 What treatment is available for vaginal trichomoniasis?

659 Tumours of the vagina are most uncommon. What are the likely pathologies?

660 What is the cause, effect and treatment of vulvovaginitis in children?

661 Why is the postmenopausal woman prone to infection?

I Diseases of the cervix

662   What is a Nabothian follicle?

663   What other benign tumour of the cervix is commonly encountered?

664   What are the symptoms and treatment of a patient with a cervical polyp?

665   What is the meaning of the term cervical erosion?

666   What symptoms may occur in a patient with a cervical erosion?

667   What treatment is required in a patient with a cervical erosion?

668   Who was Papanicolaou?

669   Who should have a cervical (Pap) smear and how often?

670   What is cervical cytology?

671   What do you understand by dyskaryosis?

672   What do you understand by the terms dysplasia and carcinoma *in situ*?

673   How are the results of cervical cytology graded?

674   This terminology has recently been modified. What is the new terminology?

675   What is the natural history of dysplasia and carcinoma *in situ*?

676   What effect does mass cervical screening programmes have on the incidence of invasive cancer of the cervix?

677   What is colposcopy?

678   Describe what is known as the transformation zone on the cervix?

679   What is an atypical transformation zone?

680 How would you manage a patient with a dyskaryotic or positive smear?

681 What methods of treatment are available to a patient with carcinoma *in situ* of the cervix?

682 What is the place of cone biopsy in the management of such patients?

683 What are the hazards of cone biopsy?

684 What is the indication for hysterectomy in the treatment of carcinoma *in situ*?

685 Why are more conservative measures now being adopted in the treatment of CIN III lesions?

686 What are the advantages of carbon dioxide laser therapy?

687 How would you deal with an 'abnormal' cervical smear in pregnancy?

688 What effect does pregnancy have on carcinoma *in situ*?

689 Does the mode of delivery have any bearing on the disease?

690 What is the commonest malignant tumour in the genital tract?

691 What epidemiological factors are associated with cervical cancer?

692 What histological types of carcinoma of the cervix are encountered?

693 How does carcinoma of the cervix commonly present?

694 What is the mode of spread of cervical cancer?

695 What are the different clinical stages of carcinoma of the cervix?

696 Briefly outline the treatment of invasive carcinoma of the cervix.

697　What are the advantages of surgical treatment of carcinoma of the cervix?

698　What are the disadvantages of surgical treatment of carcinoma of the cervix?

J　Diseases of the uterus

699　What is an endometrial polyp?

700　What forms of endometrial hyperplasia are there?

701　How is a patient with endometrial hyperplasia managed?

702　What is the correct term for a fibroid and what are its features?

703　Where, in the uterus, are fibroids found?

704　What sort of changes can occur in a fibroid?

705　What symptoms are associated with fibroids?

706　What treatment, if any, is required for uterine fibroids?

707　A patient of 45 has a midline swelling arising from the pelvis equivalent in size to a 16 week pregnancy. She is asymptomatic and is not pregnant. How would you manage the case?

708　What is the most common malignant pathology of the body of the uterus?

709　What aetiological factors are known about endometrial carcinoma?

710　How does endometrial carcinoma present?

711　How is carcinoma of the endometrium staged?

712　How is Stage I carcinoma of the endometrium treated?

713　How are later stages of the disease treated?

714 What is the prognosis for the disease?

K Diseases of the fallopian tubes

715 How may salpingitis occur?

716 What are the causes and presenting features of acute salpingitis?

717 What pathological changes occur with an acute ascending salpingitis?

718 With what other conditions may acute salpingitis be confused?

719 How do you treat acute salpingitis?

720 In postabortal and puerperal salpingitis, what are the organisms commonly involved?

721 What are the features of chronic pelvic infection?

722 What are the clinical findings in chronic pelvic infection?

723 What treatment is available for chronic pelvic infection?

724 With what other conditions can chronic pelvic infection be confused?

725 What is the incidence of pelvic tuberculosis?

726 What are the clinical features of pelvic tuberculosis?

727 What pathological findings may you find in pelvic tuberculosis?

728 How may the diagnosis of pelvic tuberculosis be made?

729 What treatment should be carried out for tuberculous salpingitis?

730 What is a hydatid of Morgagni?

731 How may carcinoma of the fallopian tube present?

L   Diseases of the ovaries

732   What are the main components of the ovary from which tumours may develop?

733   Cysts of the ovary can be neoplastic or functional. How would you describe a functional cyst?

734   Describe the clinical problems that may occur with a simple ovarian cyst.

735   What are the most common sources of confusion with an ovarian tumour that is palpable abdominally?

736   Small ovarian tumours are diagnosed on bimanual examination. What other conditions may give rise to similar findings?

737   When examining a patient, what measures would you take and what would you look for if you suspected an ovarian tumour?

738   Why do cases of malignant ovarian tumour present so late in the course of the disease?

739   Provide a simple classification of ovarian tumours.

740   Serous cystadenomata and mucinous cystadenomata are the most common cysts of the ovary, accounting for about 40 per cent of ovarian neoplasms. How do they differ?

741   Briefly outline the treatment of serous and mucinous cystadenomata.

742   What are the features of a benign teratoma (dermoid cyst)?

743   What is an endometrioid cystadenocarcinoma?

744   State the clinical staging of ovarian cancer in simple terms.

745   What is the distribution of malignant epithelial tumours of the ovary?

746 What are the main lines of therapy for malignant epithelial tumours of the ovary?

747 What is a Krukenberg tumour?

748 Describe Meig's syndrome.

M Endometriosis

749 What is endometriosis?

750 What are the essential features of the histology of areas of endometriosis or adenomyosis?

751 What are the clinical features of adenomyosis?

752 What treatment is available for adenomyosis?

753 What theories have been put forward to explain the occurrence of endometriosis?

754 What are the sites commonly associated with endometriosis?

755 In what group of patients would you expect to find endometriosis more common?

756 What are the presenting symptoms of endometriosis?

757 What are the physical signs associated with endometriosis?

758 What treatment is available for endometriosis?

759 What is stromal endometriosis?

N Uterine displacements, prolapse and associated urinary problems

760 Is a retroverted uterus an abnormal finding?

761 What symptoms may be caused by a retroverted uterus?

762 What is prolapse?

763 Describe the types of vaginal prolapse that occur.

764 What is a uterovaginal prolapse?

765 What predisposing factors favour prolapse?

766 Describe the symptoms of prolapse.

767 What may be done for a woman who has symptoms related to a prolapse?

768 In cases where procidentia has been present for a long time, the cervix may be ulcerated and there may be marked oedema. How are these cases managed?

769 A patient presents with urinary incontinence. What are the possible causes?

770 How is urinary continence normally maintained in the female?

771 What is stress incontinence?

772 What is the hoped for anatomical result of operations designed to relieve stress incontinence?

773 What operations are performed to alleviate stress incontinence?

774 How would you describe urge incontinence?

775 Outline the symptoms of a woman with an irritable bladder (detrusor instability)?

776 Discuss treatment of the unstable bladder.

777 Unfortunately a group of patients appear to have a mixed picture of both stress incontinence and bladder instability. What tests are of value in elucidating the nature of the complaint?

778 What is postmenopausal urethral syndrome?

O The climacteric and menopause

779 Distinguish between the menopause and the climacteric.

780 Describe the endocrine changes that occur during the climacteric.

781 What changes occur in the reproductive tract as a result of the climacteric?

782 How often do you think that women will seek medical help because of symptoms of the climacteric?

783 State the most common menopausal symptoms.

784 What other symptoms may be attributed to the climacteric?

785 Why is osteoporosis much more common in postmenopausal women than in men of a comparable age?

786 State why premenopausal women have a much lower incidence of coronary artery disease than men of the same age and why this difference is gradually eroded after the menopause?

787 What is the rationale of hormone replacement therapy (HRT)?

788 How should HRT be administered?

789 List the types of oestrogen available for HRT.

790 Why is it beneficial to give cyclical progestogens as well as oestrogens?

791 What symptomatic therapy may be given to women with menopausal symptoms in whom hormonal therapy is contraindicated?

P   Fertility control

Subfertility

792 How common is subfertility?

793 Before investigating the female partner, a semen analysis should be carried out (unless the male is of recently proven fertility). What features of a semen analysis are of importance and what is the range of normal values?

794 What can cause azoospermia?

795 If a man has oligozoospermia (a density below 20×10^6/ml) what can be done?

796 Can anything else be offered to couples where an abnormality of semen analysis exists?

797 What are the bases of investigation of the subfertile female?

798 What investigations are carried out to attempt to establish that ovulation is occurring?

799 How would you instruct a patient to record their basal body temperature?

800 What is the typical temperature pattern in an ovulatory cycle?

801 What are the problems associated with basal body temperature charts?

802 What other endocrine investigations would you carry out in addition to the plasma progesterone level?

803 How would you treat a patient whose plasma progesterone fell below 25 nmol/l on the 7th day prior to menses?

804 What are the common side effects of clomiphene?

805 What other forms of treatment are available to promote ovulation?

806 What is the postcoital test?

807 What are the features of ovulatory cervical mucus?

808 In patients with deficient midcycle cervical mucus can any treatment be given?

809 What might you suspect if no sperms are found in the cervical mucus at a postcoital test performed at the correct time of the cycle?

810 What can be offered to patients when the

postcoital test consistently shows non-motile sperms?

811 What forms of tubal patency tests are there?

812 What are their advantages and disadvantages?

813 Why can tubal occlusion occur?

814 What can be done for the patient with 'blocked tubes'?

Contraception

815 How is the efficiency of a particular method of contraception measured?

816 What hormonal methods of contraception are available?

817 What are the common minor side effects of the combined pill, especially in the first 3 months?

818 What other side effects may develop on the combined pill?

819 What would you consider to be contraindications to taking the pill?

820 How does the combined oral contraceptive work?

821 How does the progestogen-only pill work?

822 What problems are associated with the progestogen-only pill?

823 What are the failure rates associated with the combined and progestogen-only oral contraception?

824 What are the commonly used oestrogens and progestogens found in the combined pill?

825 How would you advise a patient who has forgotten one pill in the cycle?

53

826 Apart from forgetting to take the combined pill on a particular day or days, what other reasons may account for its failure?

827 Which patients are suitable for injectable steroids as a contraceptive?

828 What reversible barrier methods of contraception are available?

829 What intrauterine contraceptive devices (IUCDs) are currently available?

830 What are the contraindications to the introduction of an intrauterine contraceptive device (IUCD)?

831 What are the main complications of IUCD insertion?

832 What action would you take if the threads of an IUCD are not located?

833 What are the main advantages and disadvantages of the copper-bearing devices?

834 A 47-year-old patient, with no menstrual problems has had an inert device for 5 years. Do you think it is time for a change?

835 What is the rhythm method of contraception?

836 What are the problems with coitus interruptus as a method of contraception?

837 What are the advantages and problems with vasectomy?

838 What methods of female tubal sterilisation are available?

839 What are the contraindications to female tubal sterilisation?

3
Answers

OBSTETRICS

A   Basis of ante natal care

Physiology of reproduction

1   Conception is the fusion of the ovum and spermatozoon; otherwise known as fertilisation or impregnation.
[A:169; B:6; C:80; D:25; F:11]

2   A cell containing a haploid number of chromosomes has half the number of chromosomes of normal somatic cells. Mature germ cells (the ovum and spermatozoon) have a haploid chromosomal content (23 chromosomes) as distinguished from normal somatic cells which contain the diploid or full chromosome content (46 chromosomes). Following fertilisation between ovum and sperm, the diploid number of chromosomes is re-established.
[A:93; B:30; F:10]

3   The haploid number of chromosomes is achieved by a reduction division known as meiosis where the chromosomes become arranged in pairs. One member of each pair passes to each daughter cell, so halving the number of chromosomes in the mature germ cells. In mitosis or ordinary cell division, each chromosome divides into two and the two halves of each chromosome pass into the two daughter cells.
  The stem cells in the ovary and testis containing the normal 46 chromosomes, first divide by mitosis to produce daughter cells—primary oocytes and spermatocytes. These then undergo a meiotic reduction division to become secondary oocytes and spermatocytes containing 22 autosomal chromosomes and one sex chromosome in each cell. These divisions occur in the ovum and testis respectively.

The secondary oocyte will undergo a further mitotic division in the uterine tube, the final mature ovum still containing 23 chromosomes.

In the testis the spermatocyte also undergoes a further mitotic division to form two spermatids each with 23 chromosomes.
[A:93; B:30; F:10]

4   Once conception occurs the endometrial lining undergoes intense preparation for implantation of the fertilised ovum and becomes known as the decidua. This increased activity is a result of stimulation by oestrogen which increases the growth of the endometrium fourfold. It contains large maternal sinusoids which are penetrated by the blastocyst at implantation.
[A:122; B:5; F:15]

5   The egg is surrounded by follicular cells, cumulus öophorus, which adhere to the surface of the ovary until picked up by the fimbria of the fallopian tube. The cilia of the fimbria move the cumulus mass into the tube where peristalsis aids transport.
[B:32; D:13; F:11]

6   In the ampullary region of the fallopian tube.
[B:31; F:11]

7   Multiple cell division takes place whilst the ferti-lised egg or zygote is propelled along the fallopian tube. Within three days a solid mass of uniform cells has formed, known as the morula. A cavity now forms in the morula which becomes known as the blastocyst. At one end the cells clump together forming the inner cell mass, and the remainder are pushed to the peri-phery and this outer layer of the blastocyst becomes known as the trophoblast.
[A:103; B:32; C:82; D:15; F:13]

8   The blastocyst. This is a stage reached 5–7 days after conception.
[A:107; B:32; C:82; D:26; F:11]

9   The trophoblast differentiates into two layers: the outer syncytiotrophoblast in contact with maternal blood consisting of a multinuclear syncytium with no distinct cell boundaries; and

an inner cytotrophoblast layer of single cuboidal cells.
[A:110; B:33; C:82; D:17; F:13]

10 The inner cell mass differentiates into an outer ectodermal layer and an inner endodermal layer. A further differentiation produces a third layer—the mesoderm between these two. The opposing layers of ectoderm and endoderm and interspersed mesoderm are destined to form the embryo.
[A:112; B:33; C:82; D:17; F:13]

11 The *ectoderm* forms the nervous system including the medulla of the adrenal, and glands such as the anterior pituitary and salivary.
The *endoderm* forms the gastrointestinal tract, liver, gall bladder, biliary tract, pancreas, respiratory tract, germ cells of gonads.
The *mesoderm* forms bone, muscle, cartilage connective tissue, cardiovascular system, kidneys and most of the genital tract.
[A:112; B:33; C:82; F:13]

12 11–12 weeks. At this stage ossification centres appear in most bones.
[B:35]

13 To produce human chorionic gonadotrophin (HCG). This ensures the persistence of the corpus luteum (and hence progesterone production) until the trophoblast is capable of manufacturing sufficient quantities itself. This luteoplacental shift occurs about 4–5 weeks after conception.
[A:117; B:33; D:41; F:8]

14 The placenta is the means through which the fetus obtains its needs.
Its functions can be classified as:
(a) nutritional,
(b) respiratory,
(c) excretory,
(d) endocrine,
(e) barrier against infection and immunological rejection.
[A:147; B:38; C:86; D:33; F:20]

15 (a) Passive transport—either by simple or facilitated diffusion. The former occurs when substances move from a higher to a lower

concentration area; the latter more rapidly because of the shape and structure of the molecule.

(b) Active transport—this occurs with the transport of inorganic ions and some substrates. Enzymatic systems are required or pinocytosis may occur in which complex molecules are engulfed by microvilli.

[A:205; B:38; C:86; D:33; F:21]

Maternal physiology

16 25 per cent of the non-pregnant weight. This usually averages 12·5 kg for the whole pregnancy.
[A:310; B:60; C:121; D:51; F:40]

17 Plasma volume increases throughout pregnancy to reach a maximum by 35 weeks. Thereafter it falls slightly, with a further drop at delivery. It returns to non-pregnant levels by six weeks post partum.
[A:232; B:195; C:119; D:47; F:41]

18 The cardiac output has risen markedly (by approximately 40 per cent) by 12 weeks' gestation and continues at this increased level throughout pregnancy and increases again by approximately 15 per cent during labour.
[A:238; B:191; C:120; D:48; F:42]

19 There is a slight increase in pulse rate (about 15 per cent) but the major contribution is by a large increase in stroke volume. This is balanced by a decrease in peripheral resistance and the blood pressure alters very little.
[A:238; B:191; C:120; D:48; F:42]

20 Pressure of the gravid uterus on the inferior vena cava. This leads to diminished cardiac return and hence reduced cardiac output. The patient feels faint and may become pale and sweaty. Changes of the fetal heart rate are common.
[A:239; B:191; C:280; F:42]

21 The red cell mass is increased as a result of stimulation of erythropoiesis by increased levels of

erythropoietin and by human placental lactogen.
[A:233; C:119; F:41]

22 Fibrinogen levels increase together with platelet production. Fibrinolytic activity is reduced during pregnancy probably as a result of low levels of fibrinolytic activators.
[B:197; C:305; F:430]

23 The renal blood flow is increased (by 230 ml/min) as is the glomerular filtration rate (from 100 to 120 ml per minute) and creatinine clearance rises to between 150 and 200 ml/min.
[A:241; B:214; C:122, 319; D:50]

24 There is an increase in the tidal volume due to deeper respiration. The respiratory rate is not increased. There is a lowered arterial Pco_2. These changes are probably caused by progesterone affecting the respiratory centres
[A:240; B:190; C:121; D:49; F:42]

25 (a) The gums become swollen and bleed more easily.
(b) Excessive salivation may occur (ptyalism).
(c) Heartburn (reflux oesophagitis) is common from 12 weeks onwards. It is often exacerbated by lying flat in late pregnancy.
(d) The stomach tends to empty more slowly, particularly in labour.
(e) Constipation—this may be due to slowing of peristalsis, obstructive effect of the gravid uterus in late pregnancy, poor diet, oral iron therapy.
(f) Fissure-in-ano. Probably the result of passing hard faecal material.
[A:247; B:205; C:122; F:43]

Anatomy

26 Four types of pelvis are described—gynaecoid (55 per cent), android (20 per cent), anthropoid (20 per cent) and platypelloid (5 per cent).
   In the gynaecoid pelvis the brim is almost round. In the android pelvis the brim is heart-shaped due to a projecting sacral promontory and narrow forepelvis. The anthropoid pelvic brim is oval and also tends to have midpelvic

narrowing. The platypelloid brim is transversely oval with usually a shallow pelvis and capacious outlet.
[A:286; B:313; F:296]

27   It is heart-shaped, narrowing anteriorly. The subpelvic arch is reduced, often less than 90° and the ischial spines prominent. The *available* space at the brim is reduced, even though the anteroposterior diameter may be greater than that of a gynaecoid pelvis.
[A:287; D:333; F:297]

28   The superior aspects of the pubic bones, the ileopectineal eminences and lines, the ala and promontory of the sacrum. In the gynaecoid pelvis the brim is almost round.
[A:275; B:20; D:77]

29   The obstetric conjugate is the available diameter for passage of the fetal head through the pelvic brim and is measured from the sacral promontory to the nearest point on the posterior surface of the symphysis pubis and measures approximately 11·5 cm. The diagonal conjugate can be measured clinically from the lower border of the symphysis pubis to the promontory of the sacrum (12·5 cm) and is used to assess the anteroposterior diameter of the pelvic brim. The anatomical or true conjugate is the measurement from the sacral promontory to the upper border of the symphysis pubis.
[A:278; B:23; D:81]

30   The vertex is the area bounded by the anterior and posterior fontanelle and laterally by the two parietal eminences.
[A:295; B:11; D:92; F:85]

31   95 per cent of babies are born by the vertex.
[A:296]

32   The biparietal diameter is the distance between the parietal eminences and measures approximately 9·5 cm at term. In a vertex presentation it is the largest presenting diameter.
[A:176; B:25; D:93]

33   The pelvic floor is comprised of the levator ani muscles which run from the symphisis pubis

anteriorly, around the lateral pelvic wall to the ischial spine and the coccyx. The floor is completed by fascial condensations on its upper and lower surfaces and is pierced by the urethra, vagina and rectum. It is gutter-shaped, running forwards and downwards. This aids flexion and anterior rotation of the fetal head as it descends through the pelvis.
[B:24; D:85; F:83]

Diagnosis of pregnancy

34 Early symptoms of pregnancy are missed period, nausea, weight gain, breast tenderness and urinary frequency. None of these or only some are necessarily present in every patient.
[A:270; B:41; D:53; F:45]

35 The breasts are fuller and superficial veins often prominent. Montgomery's tubercles around the nipple are enlarged. The cervix takes on a purplish colour and the uterus is soft, globular and enlarged. Arterial pulsations are often felt in the lateral fornices.
[A:261; B:41; D:53; F:46]

36 Chloasma. Its probable cause is an increased pituitary output of melanocyte stimulating hormone (MSH).
[A:228; B:183; C:118; F:44]

37 Pregnancy tests are dependent on the production of human chorionic gonadotrophin (HCG) secreted 14 days after fertilisation by the blastocyst. A peak is reached at 10–12 weeks and the hormone is excreted in the mother's urine.
[A:267; B:41; C:125; D:54; F:49]

38 The pregnancy test usually becomes negative at 16–18 weeks gestation when HCG levels fall.
      Tests may remain positive for at least two days following abortion.
[F:50]

39 Fetal movements are first felt at approximately 18–20 weeks in primigravid patients and slightly earlier at 16–18 weeks in multigravida.
[A:262; B:149; D:55; F:47]

40   Fetal parts can first be palpated at approximately
      24–26 weeks' gestation.
      [A:265; D:55; F:47]

Ante natal care

41   (a) To monitor the well-being of the fetus
          throughout pregnancy.
      (b) To establish and maintain the physical
          health of the mother.
      (c) To give psychological support to the expect-
          ant mother.
      (d) To provide an opportunity for the mother to
          familiarise herself with the staff who are
          going to care for her and the environment
          into which she is going to bring her baby.
      [A:303; B:43; C:124; D:58; F:54]

42   A primiparous patient is one who has delivered
      one viable baby, or a stillbirth after 28 completed
      weeks of pregnancy. A primigravid patient is
      one who is pregnant for the first time. A patient
      may therefore be multigravid (i.e. had a number
      of abortions, spontaneous or otherwise) and still
      be primiparous or nulliparous.
          It is the number of pregnancies reaching
      viability and not the number of fetuses delivered
      that determines parity (i.e. delivering twins or
      triplets does not increase parity).
      [A:304; B:6]

43   Ideally before 14 weeks. At this stage an accurate
      assessment of uterine size can be made; various
      screening procedures arranged or carried out
      (e.g. ultrasound examination, α-fetoprotein
      levels etc.); amniocentesis arranged if necessary;
      the cervix assessed for incompetence; and early
      assessment of maternal health made etc.
      [A:305; B:43; D:64]

44   After the initial visit to the hospital, the patient
      should be seen monthly until 28 weeks preg-
      nant, at 2-weekly intervals until 36 weeks and
      thereafter weekly unless her condition warrants
      more frequent visits. In the UK, the visits are
      most often shared between the hospital and the
      family doctor who has a particular interest in
      obstetrics.
      [A:308; B:47; D:65; F:56]

45 At the first ante natal visit, a full history should include:
   (a) age; first day of LMP; menstrual cycle and marital status;
   (b) relevant past medical or surgical history;
   (c) previous obstetric history to include birth weight, sex, gestation, length of labour, type of delivery;
   (d) relevant family and social history to determine in particular the presence or absence of congenital abnormalities, diabetes, multiple pregnancy, tuberculosis and also to enquire about smoking and alcohol consumption.
   [A:306; B:43; D:64; F:54]

46 (a) Examination to include height, weight, blood pressure and urinalysis.
   (b) A general examination to assess the patient's general health, cardiovascular and respiratory systems.
   (c) Examination of the breasts and abdomen— include assessment of uterine size if possible.
   (d) Examination of the legs for varicosities and/or oedema.
   (e) A vaginal and bimanual examination.
   [A:307; B:44; F:55]

47 A vaginal and bimanual examination carried out at the first ante natal visit not only can confirm the diagnosis of pregnancy and assess uterine size accurately, but also excludes other pelvic abnormalities such as fibroids, ovarian or vaginal cysts, retroversion, bicornuate uterus and vaginal septa. It also allows one to inspect the vulva for varicosities and condylomata and to take a cervical smear and high vaginal swab, if necessary.
   With the advent of routine ultrasound screening the necessity to perform bimanual examination is considerably lessened.
   [B:45; C:125; F:56]

48 A vaginal examination should be omitted at the first ante natal visit if there has been a history of recent bleeding or of repeated miscarriages.

49 (a) Blood grouping (A B O and rhesus).
   (b) Abnormal antibody titres.

    (c) Haemaglobin.
    (d) Serological tests for syphilis.
    (e) Rubella antibody titre.
    (f) Serum α-fetoprotein estimation is performed between 16 and 19 weeks as a routine in many clinics in the UK.
[A:306; B:47; D:65; F:55]

50   At each ante natal visit, urine is tested for protein and sugar; the patient is weighed; the blood pressure recorded. Observations about bleeding or reduced fetal movements are recorded. Clinical examination will assess uterine growth, presentation of the fetus and the presence or absence of oedema.
[B:52; D:65]

51   The presence of protein in routine urine testing may be a result of contaminants. Repeat testing of a midstream specimen of urine is always indicated. Protein will be found in urine which contains vaginal discharge, blood, pus or liquor amnii, and also in the event of a urinary tract infection. Protein may also be found as a late manifestation of hypertension of pregnancy and in eclampsia, chronic renal disease, hyperemesis gravidarum and cardiac disease.
[B:54]

52   Blood pressure recordings in pregnancy of 140/90 and over or an increase in systolic blood pressure greater than 30 mmHg or diastolic blood pressure greater than 15 mmHg, over that recorded at the first ante natal visit, can be regarded as abnormal because perinatal mortality rates rise in association with such increases.
[A:666; B:193; D:66]

53   It may lead to hypertension, pre-eclampsia and intrauterine growth retardation. It will also be a lot harder to lose after pregnancy! Remember that in the very obese, falsely high blood pressure readings may be obtained because of the large girth of the arm and the relatively small width of the cuff of the sphygmomanometer. Appropriate adjustments should be made.
[B:52; C:130; D:51; F:187]

54   The significance of weight gain in pregnancy is

such that there is a high correlation between static or falling weight and the occurrence of light-for-dates babies.
[A:310; C:130; D:51]

55 Bleeding in the mid trimester of pregnancy is associated with a considerable increase in perinatal mortality and light-for-dates infants.

56 There is mounting evidence that smoking in pregnancy leads to intrauterine growth retardation. There is a higher incidence of premature labour in women who smoke and the overall perinatal mortality is increased. It appears that it is the carbon monoxide in the inhaled smoke that is largely responsible for these problems.
[A:320; B:57; D:74; F:65]

57 In the healthy woman with an uncomplicated obstetric history and pregnancy, there is no restriction on coitus right up to term. However, in patients who have threatened to abort, who have a previous history of premature labour, who have had an ante partum haemorrhage or where the membranes are thought to have ruptured, restrictions on sexual activity should be imposed.
[A:319; B:56; D:74; F:59]

58 It is caused by reflux of gastric contents into the lower oesophagus. Relaxation of the cardiac 'sphincter', the effect of progesterone on smooth muscle, the supine position, smoking, and the pressure effect of the enlarging uterus all contribute to the condition. It can occur as early as 12 weeks' gestation and is seen in over 60 per cent of patients.
[A:324; B:62; D:175; F:43]

59 The patient should be advised to take small frequent meals, smoking should be reduced or preferably stopped and three pillows used in bed. Antacids are often of considerable use.
[B:63; D:175]

60 All patients experience an increase in leucorrhoea due to the high oestrogen state and increase in mucus secretion from the cervix. Fungal infections are common, causing intense itching and a heavy creamy non-offensive

discharge. Trichomonal infections cause a greenish, frothy and very offensive discharge. In both cases the patient and her sexual partner should be treated. Foreign bodies in the vagina such as a cervical suture or Hodge pessary will also increase the discharge.
[A:325; C:364; D:182; F:62]

61 The patient should be taught how to evert the nipples herself from about 28 weeks onwards. The wearing of nipple shields inside the brassière will usually improve the condition.
[B:413; F:60]

62 Varicose veins in pregnancy are caused by decreased tone in the vessels leading to dilatation and increased pressure on the pelvic veins leading to decreased venous return from the lower limbs. The condition is exacerbated in the standing position.
[A:323; B:63; D:177; F:62]

63 Abdominal palpation in the latter half of pregnancy reveals:
(a) the fundal height;
(b) the lie of the fetus—longitudinal, oblique or transverse;
(c) the presentation of fetus—cephalic or breech;
(d) whether the presenting part is engaged;
(e) size of the fetus;
(f) presence of abnormal conditions such as polyhydramnios, multiple pregnancy or abdominal tumours.
[F:100]

64 The fingers of the right hand are placed suprapubically and grasp the fetal head. The thumb and the middle finger are the important palpating digits. Remember that the lower segment is more sensitive than the upper and this is a painful examination if performed without the maximum of gentleness. If you need to do it in a clinical examination, ask the patient to tell you if it is uncomfortable. This shows respect for the patient, is good manners (and may earn you an extra mark!)
[A:298; B:49; D:69; F:103]

65 Engagement has occurred when the widest diameter of the presenting part has passed through

the pelvic brim (vide supra). (This is one of the most commonly used terms in obstetrics, is frequently asked by examiners and seldom answered correctly by examinees.)
[A:282; B:50; D:70; F:102]

66   (a) Full bladder ⎫ possibly the most common.
     (b) Full rectum ⎭
     (c) Placenta praevia—the most sinister.
     (d) Pelvic tumour—fibroid, ovarian cyst, double uterus.
     (e) 'Cephalopelvic disproportion'.
     (f) Posterior position of fetal head.
     (g) Multiple pregnancy.
     (h) Breech presentation.
     (i) Polyhydramnios.
     (j) Grand multiparity.
     (k) Racial—non-engagement is very common in West Africans.
     (l) Misdiagnosis of gestational age (i.e. prematurity).
     (m) Uterine anomalies.
     (n) Hydrocephaly.
     [B:52; D:70]

67   The indications for lateral pelvimetry are diminishing. It is quite wrong to assume that you can assess the ability of a baby's head to pass through the birth canal by sitting in a darkened room and staring at an X-ray film. The diagnosis of disproportion can only be made by allowing the patient to go into labour. It depends not only on the size of the baby's head and the shape of the pelvis but also on the position of the head, its degree of flexion and efficient uterine action.
     [A:285; B:84; F:105]

Uterine displacements and anomalies

68   Most of these tumours represent a corpus luteum cyst and removal at this stage could lead to abortion, despite the fact that the luteoplacental shift of function has probably taken place by now. The patient should be re-examined at 12 weeks. If the cyst is the same size or bigger it should be removed before the 16th week of pregnancy because of the risk of torsion rupture, haemorrhage or obstruction.
     [A:851; B:219; C:762; F:246]

69   Operative intervention at this stage is not advisable. If the cyst becomes impacted in the pelvis, vaginal delivery will not be possible and caesarean section will be necessary (at which time the cyst can be removed). If the tumour does not obstruct labour, then laparotomy should be undertaken in the puerperium.
      [A:855; B:220; C:763; D:266; F:248]

70   Incarceration of the retroverted gravid uterus. In this condition the cervix is displaced upwards stretching the urethra until a time is reached when voiding becomes impossible. Treatment is urethral catheterisation for 48 hours, in which time the uterus usually 'escapes' from the pelvis. Manual anteversion is not recommended.
      [A:633; B:217; C:365; F:241]

71   The possible effects of fibroids are early or late abortion, premature labour, unstable lie, non-engagement of the fetal head and obstructed labour. However, the effects depend entirely upon the size and position of the tumour. Small or subserous fibroids seldom have any effect.
      [A:850; B:219; C:702; D:264; F:243]

72   If the myoma is lying in the pelvis, labour may become obstructed and caesarean section necessary. Otherwise, they do not alter the quality of the contractions. Fibroids that distort the cavity of the uterus may lead to post partum haemorrhage. Myomectomy should never be undertaken during pregnancy or at the time of a caesarean section.
      [A:850; D:265]

73   (a) Faults in the fusion of the two Müllerian ducts may lead to a double vagina, double cervix or double uterus. Minor faults of the uterus are more common (such as arcuate and subseptate uterus or bicornuate uterus).
      (b) Faults in the development of one duct will give rise to unicornuate uterus or incomplete elements of one side (e.g. rudimentary horn).
      (c) Faulty canalisation of one or both of the ducts. This can lead to an absent vagina or haematometra. Occluding membranes of the vagina are more common and are a cause

of primary amenorrhoea and haematocolpos.
[A:627; B:218; C:6; D:181; F:243]

74 Abortion and premature labour are four times as common. Malpresentations such as breech and transverse lie are also more common. In cases of double uterus, the non-pregnant uterus may obstruct the descent of the fetal head and caesarean section becomes necessary.
[A:627; B:218; C:215; D:181; F:243; I:256]

B   Assessment of fetal well-being

Amniocentesis, prenatal diagnosis and genetics

75 Estimation of maternal serum α-fetoprotein levels between 16 and 18 weeks' gestation is a screening procedure for open neural tube defects. Assessment of gestational age must be accurate as levels vary widely with differing gestational ages. Raised levels indicate the possibility of an affected fetus.
[A:343; B:136; C:786; D:446; D:370]

76 There is a relatively high false positive rate leading to unnecessary amniocentesis in healthy pregnancies (and resultant abortion in a few). The levels may be raised following threatened abortion. The test will not reveal closed neural tube defects.
[A:343]

77 Raised serum AFP levels can also be associated with exomphalos and congenital nephrosis. It is also raised in twin pregnancies, threatened abortion and maternal liver disease.
[A:343]

78 Raised serum AFP levels are an indication to suspect intrauterine growth retardation. Approximately 1 in 7 patients with raised serum AFP will deliver a low birth weight infant.

79 It is suggested that the incidence of neural tube defects can be reduced by prescribing multivitamins three times daily for 3 months prior to conception and for the first 2 months of pregnancy.

80   For the diagnosis of suspected chromosomal abnormalities of the fetus; to assess the α-feto-protein (AFP) levels when a neural tube defect is suspected (e.g. raised maternal α-fetoprotein or very strong history); to measure bile pigments in cases of rhesus isoimmunisation; to promote a therapeutic abortion using hypertonic solutions with or without prostaglandins; fetoscopy.
[A:330; B:134]

81   Amniocentesis should be carried out between 16 and 18 weeks' gestation.
[A:330; B:135; C:787; F:369]

82   Information obtained from aspirating amniotic fluid in the second and third trimester of pregnancy is of value in assessment of:
(a) cytogenetics,
(b) fetal ageing,
(c) rhesus disease,
(d) AFP levels (neural tube defects).
[A:330; B:134; C:401; F:369]

83   The dangers of amniocentesis are: rupture of the membranes; abortion (1–2 per cent); fetal death *in utero*; fetal damage; infection; rhesus isoimmunisation.
[A:330; B:134; C:401; F:369]

84   Hereditary and biochemical disorders may be identified from cell culture following amniocentesis. These cells retain their enzyme activity and a number of diseases have been identified such as:
(a) disorders of lipid metabolism—Tay–Sachs, Gaucher and Niemann–Pick disease;
(b) disorders of carbohydrate metabolism—galactosaemia;
(c) disorders of mucopolysaccharide metabolism—Hurler's and Hunter's syndromes;
(d) disorders of amino acid metabolism—maple syrup urine disease.
[A:340]

85   The most common chromosomal abnormality seen at birth is trisomy-21 (Down's syndrome). The overall incidence is 1 : 630 but there is a marked increase when the mother's age exceeds 40.
[A:996; C:785]

86   The incidence of Down's syndrome (trisomy-21) increases with maternal age. At the age of 35 the risk is in the order of 1 in 360 pregnancies. At the age of 40 the risk is 1 in 80 and at 44 years of age a 1 in 40 chance of an affected infant.
      [A:996; C:785]

87   If both parents carry a recessive gene, one in four children will be affected (homozygous), two out of four will be carriers of the recessive gene (heterozygous) and one in four will be un-affected.
      [B:100; C:778]

88   If a female is carrying a sex-linked abnormal gene, two out of four children will be affected (the male will suffer clinically, the female will be a carrier). The affected male can only produce normal males or carrier females.
      [B:100]

89   Non-disjunction occurs when a chromosome does not separate and one of its daughter cells therefore has no chromosome of its type whereas the other daughter cell has two.
      [A:102; B:102]

90   Translocation occurs when part of one chromosome becomes attached to another.
      [B:101; C:780]

91   Examples of dominantly inherited genetic disorders are: Huntington's chorea; osteogenesis imperfecta; Marfan's syndrome; cleft palate; polycystic kidneys.
      [B:103]

92   Examples of X-linked recessive disorders are: Duchenne's muscular dystrophy, mucopolysaccharidosis and haemophilia.
      [B:103]

Assessment of gestational age

93   Add seven days to the date of the first day of the last menstrual period and deduct three calendar months. (Note: this is only correct if the patient has a regular 28 day cycle.)
      [D:64; F:52]

94 (a) An irregular cycle.
    (b) A regular cycle in excess of 28 days (e.g. 35 or 42 days).
    (c) Conception occurring after stopping the oral contraceptive pill and prior to the onset of normal menses.
    (d) Decidual haemorrhage—this form of bleeding often differs from a normal menstrual period and may not occur at precisely the correct time for a normal period. Therefore take a careful history.
    (e) Patient poor memory.
    [F:52]

95 (a) In the first trimester by bimanual examination of the uterus. This is the most accurate time to assess uterine size.
    (b) By noting the date of 'quickening' (i.e. the first time the patient is aware of fetal movement). It occurs approximately five calendar months prior to the EDD.
    (c) Ultrasound examination of the fetal biparietal diameter up to 24 weeks' gestation. After this time the standard deviation is too great for accurate dating of the pregnancy.
    (d) When faced with the problem in the third trimester clinical judgement and radiology are both notoriously inaccurate. If induction is contemplated, then lung maturity should be assessed using the lecithin/sphingomyelin ratio test (LSR).
    [F:52]

96 Incorrect dates, multiple pregnancy, uterine tumours (e.g. fibroids), trophoblastic disease, a full bladder, a full rectum. The last two are probably the most common causes and the most commonly forgotten. Also, early in the second trimester, the fundus may be higher than usual in patients who have had a previous caesarean section and in certain ethnic groups (especially West Africans and West Indians).
    [B:52]

97 Tests available for assessment of fetal maturity in the third trimester are:
    (a) radiology. This depends upon the radiological appearance of certain epiphyses—notably the lower end of femur and upper

end of tibia. These appear between 36 and 40 weeks and their presence indicates a mature infant. However, in cases of intrauterine growth retardation their appearance may be delayed even in a very mature (but small) infant. Conversely it may be hastened in diabetic pregnancies.

(b) amniotic fluid examination.

(i) Nile blue sulphate test. This substance stains fetal fat-filled cells orange and a total count of greater than 20 per cent indicates a maturity of greater than 36 weeks. It is inaccurate and of little clinical importance nowadays.

(ii) creatinine concentration—if the levels exceed 2·0 mg/100 ml, the fetus is likely to be of more than 36 weeks' gestation. However, the converse is not true especially in intrauterine growth retardation. The test has little clinical value nowadays.

(iii) lecithin sphyngomyelin ratio (LSR) If the ratio of lecithin is more than 2·0 to sphyngomyelin, it is highly unlikely that respiratory distress syndrome will develop. It is the most useful clinical test and is now widely used.

[A:329; B:149; C:128; D:277; F:52]

98 The two rises in the LSR that occur are caused by two separate biosynthetic pathways. The major pathway occurs at 34 weeks with the production of dipalmitoyl lecithin. At 28 weeks, there is a short-lived production of another phospholipid (α-methyl β-cresyl lecithin).

99 A fetus with a mature LSR may develop respiratory distress syndrome if:
(a) the mother has diabetes mellitus.
(b) the mother suffers from rhesus isoimmunisation.
(c) severe acute hypoxic states occur in labour.
[A:334]

100 Radiological signs of fetal death are gas in the great vessels, overlapping of the cranial bones (Spalding's sign), and a collapsed fetus, notably a marked flexion of the spine.
[A:272; B:148; C:151; D:194; F:108]

101 Primary placental dysfunction leads to poor implantation and nutritional deprivation of the embryo usually resulting in abortion. On occasions the fetus survives but fails to thrive *in utero* and a low birth weight baby is born with a small placenta.

Secondary placental dysfunction may arise in association with acute hypertension of pregnancy and renal disease. Spasm of the aterioles reduces placental blood flow and oxygenation of the fetus.

The fetus in pregnancies affected by primary or secondary placental dysfunction is said to suffer from intrauterine growth retardation (IUGR).
[B:141; D:279; F:250]

102 The common causes of placental dysfunction in pregnancy are:
  (a) prolonged hypertensive disease of pregnancy;
  (b) chronic renal conditions;
  (c) prolonged pregnancy;
  (d) severe anaemia;
  (e) placental abruption;
  (f) severe maternal pyrexia;
  (g) maternal diabetes (with renal involvement).
[B:142; D:279; F:250]

103 There are two groups of patients who require monitoring for IUGR:
  (a) those with a past history of a stillbirth, bad obstetric history or those with a complicating factor known to be associated with IUGR;
  (b) those whose pregnancies appear to be normal but where the fetus is suffering from intrauterine malnutrition—this group will produce half of all the growth retarded pregnancies.
[A:9, 42; B:141; D:280]

104 Clinical parameters that can be of help in assessing intrauterine growth retardation are:
  (a) maternal weight gain—static or falling weight has a significant association with IUGR. Patients beginning pregnancy weighing less than 53 kilograms and gaining

less than 5 kilograms in weight are also at high risk of producing a light-for-dates infant.

(b) uterine volume—crude assessment by measuring fundal height and girth measurements can be useful in predicting IUGR.

(c) vaginal bleeding—a history of vaginal bleeding in the second trimester results in a considerably increased incidence of peri-natal mortality and light-for-dates infants.

105 IUGR has the following effect on post natal growth and development of the baby:

(a) the neonatal mortality rate is four times that of infants of normal weight;

(b) infants more than two standard deviations below the mean have an 18 per cent inci-dence of mental retardation;

(c) 25 per cent of growth retarded babies have speech aberrations persisting into school age.

106 The increased mortality and morbidity from IUGR can be reduced by:

(a) ante natal detection;

(b) ante natal fetal monitoring;

(c) correct timing of delivery.

[A:942; B:414; D:280]

Ante partum tests

107 Methods currently available for assessing fetal well-being are:

(a) fetal movements,

(b) ultrasound,

(c) human placental lactogen (HPL),

(d) urinary and plasma oestrogens,

(e) ante natal cardiotocography,

(f) fetal breathing movements.

[A:329; B:143; C:147; D:280; F:56; I:106, 125, 1020]

108 Present evidence suggests that if less than ten movements are felt in any 12 hour period, there is a significantly raised fetal mortality. Patients are encouraged to report such a reduction in movements to their obstetrician or hospital

clinic immediately. Unstressed cardiotoco-graphy should be carried out and the appro-priate action taken dependant upon the results.
[A:348; B:143; C:129; F:252]

109 The uses of ultrasound scanning in the second trimester of pregnancy are:
   (a) to assess fetal gestational age by measuring the biparietal diameter. The earlier it is per-formed in the second trimester, the more accurate the assessment. After 24 weeks the standard deviation becomes too great.
   (b) in the diagnosis of fetal abnormality, parti-cularly anencephaly and spina bifida.
   (c) for the localisation of the placenta prior to amniocentesis.
   (d) for the diagnosis of trophoblastic disease.
   (e) for the diagnosis of multiple pregnancy.
   [A:345; B:143; C:153; D:165; F:111; I:1016]

110 The important uses of ultrasound in the third trimester are:
   (a) to assess fetal growth rate. Serial biparietal measurements are of particular use in 'at risk pregnancies' where intrauterine growth retardation is suspected. It is quite pointless to measure the biparietal diameter for the first time at 38 weeks' gestation.
   (b) for the serial monitoring of placental posi-tion in patients with suspected placenta praevia. The placenta may appear to 'move up' the uterus because of uterine differential growth.
   (c) to exclude placenta praevia in cases of ante partum haemorrhage.
   (d) ante natal monitoring using cardiotoco-graphy.

111 The ratio of head to abdominal circumference appears to be more successful at diagnosing IUGR. The brain is the last organ to be effected in growth retardation and fall off in growth of the fetal skull is a late sign. The ratio of head circum-ference (at the level of the third ventricle) and abdominal circumference (at the level of the um-bilical vein) can detect IUGR at an earlier stage.
[A:345; C:153; I:1030]

112 Human placental lactogen (HPL) produced by

the syncytotrophoblast reflects placental function. Levels below $4\,\mu g$/ml after 35 weeks' gestation indicates fetal jeopardy. Low levels of HPL are associated with low birth weight babies.
[C:161; I:106, 128]

113 Oestriol estimation is the only biochemical assessment of the fetoplacental unit. Other tests are of placental function alone. However, there are very wide standard deviations and diurnal variations and only trends are significant (i.e. single measurements unless below the standard deviation are valueless).
[A:159; B:144; C:156; D:282; F:57; I:127]

114 Total oestrogen concentrations can be affected by: maternal liver disease; antibiotic therapy (e.g. ampicillin) and steroids and impaired renal function which may reduce oestrogen concentration in plasma and urine.
[A:159; C:157; D:283; I:127]

115 Hormone assays in assessment of fetal wellbeing may not be entirely reliable in that clearance rates differ from patient to patient, and biological and technical variations can result in large falls in levels which are not pathologically significant. Fetal death *in utero* has also been encountered before placental function tests become abnormal.
[A:149; C:156; I:126]

116 Cardiotocography is a continual recording of the fetal heart rate and uterine activity. The fetal heart rate can be monitored internally by the application of a scalp electrode (only after membrane rupture) or externally via an ultrasound transducer.

117 Response of the fetal heart rate to uterine contractions produced by oxytocic stimulation is known as a stress test. Many people now regard this form of assessment as dangerous when fetal compromise is already suspected. Ante natal unstressed cardiotocography—response of the fetal heart rate to Braxton Hicks contractions—is now the generally preferred method of assessing fetal well-being.
[A:349]

118 The advantage of ante natal unstressed cardiotocography with correct interpretation gives up to the minute information on fetal well-being. However, fetal deaths *in utero* have been observed on rare occasions to occur within 24 hours of a normal recording.
[A:352; B:145; C:165]

119 The recording should be for at least 20 minutes, there must be maternally observed fetal activity and a spontaneous uterine contraction should be present. The fetal heart baseline rate should be between 120 and 160 beats per minute, there must be baseline variability (beat-to-beat variation) and the tracing should be reactive (i.e. accelerations of heart rate occurring with fetal movements or uterine contractions).
[A:345; C:167; D:281]

120 Fetal breathing patterns seen on real-time ultrasound have revealed that the occurrence of a mixed pattern of deep prolonged chest wall movements interspersed with episodes of normal breathing activity and long periods of apnoea are prognostic signs of fetal jeopardy. Deep prolonged chest movements and periods of apnoea suggest a severely compromised fetus in imminent danger of intrauterine death.
[C:165]

Intrapartum monitoring

121 Methods available for monitoring uterine contractions are:
(a) palpation;
(b) external tocometry—pressure transducer over uterine fundus;
(c) internal tocometry—fluid-filled catheter within the amniotic cavity connected to a manometer. This is the only method capable of measuring resting tone and intensity of contractions.
All three measure duration and frequency.
[A:354; F:314; I:563]

122 Clinically this is recognised by the presence of a fetal tachycardia or bradycardia and/or the appearance of meconium in the liquor. It represents fetal hypoxia or acidosis. There are a

variety of patterns seen on a cardiotocograph that represent varying degrees of fetal distress.
[A:355; B:306; C:167; D:287; F:351; I:580]

123 The methods available for monitoring fetal heart rate are:
(a) intermittent auscultation.
(b) continuous recording
(i) phonocardiography. A microphone is strapped to mother's abdomen but the quality of recording is influenced by the intensity of fetal heart sounds, fetal movements and extraneous sounds; poor recording during contractions may occur.
(ii) ultrasound. An external transducer is strapped to mother's abdomen and employs the Doppler shift principle; the fetal heart movements are complex, therefore considerable electronic damping is required. Erroneous recordings of beat-to-beat variations may occur.
(iii) fetal scalp electrode. The electrode is attached to the presenting part of the fetus and therefore the membranes must be ruptured. The rate is computed by measurement of the time interval between two successive R waves. It is uninfluenced by maternal or fetal movement.
[A:353; B:307; C:267; D:276; F:352; I:581]

124 A normal fetal heart rate pattern in labour has the following characteristics.
(a) normal baseline rate 120–160 beats per minute;
(b) no significant change of baseline rate during contractions; except accelerations;
(c) good beat-to-beat variation.
[A:355; B:307; C:167; D:287; F:354; I:582]

125 Beat-to-beat variation is a phenomenon noted on cardiotocograph tracings. In the healthy fetus, it represents dynamic governing of the fetal heart rate by the autonomic nervous system and should exceed eight beats. If the variation is less then five beats the fetus may be compromised. External monitoring can be unreliable because faulty positioning of the ultrasound transducer may lead to erroneous variability.
[A:357; B:235; C:167; D:287]

126 In interpretation of the FHR pattern, the following abnormalities may be observed:
(a) fetal bradycardia;
(b) fetal tachycardia;
(c) loss of baseline irregularity;
(d) early deceleration or type 1 dip;
(e) late deceleration or type 2 dip;
(f) variable decelerations;
(g) dip area.
[A:355; B:307; C:167; D:288; F:352; I:582]

127 Baseline bradycardia is a FHR of less than 120 beats per minute. If associated with other abnormalities, it is an adverse sign.
[A:357; B:307; C:167; F:353; I:583]

128 Baseline tachycardia is a FHR greater than 160 beats per minute. It may herald fetal hypoxia or reflect maternal excitement, dehydration or pyrexia.
[A:357; B:307; C:167; F:353; I:583]

129 It is a synchronous or early deceleration of the fetal heart rate during a contraction. It is usually due to head compression and vagal reflex activity with an amplitude of usually less than 40 beats per minute. It is normally of no significance but may be an early sign of cord compression or hypoxia due to placental insufficiency. If the pattern deteriorates into variable or late decelerations, further investigation is necessary.
[A:356; B:307; C:167; D:288; F:355; I:582]

130 It is a late deceleration of fetal heart rate occurring at least 20 seconds after the onset of a contraction. The deceleration may be as little as 15 beats and is often associated with loss of baseline variability and a tachycardia which is a most ominous pattern. It is associated with fetal hypoxia and suggests placental insufficiency. It may be a sign of impending fetal death.
[A:356; B:307; C:167; D:288; F:356; I:582]

131 These are decelerations that have a variable onset and depth. Their significance depends upon the baseline rate and variability and the stage of labour at which they occur. Umbilical cord compression is a common cause and the

abnormality may be corrected by changes in maternal position.
[A:356; B:307; C:167; D:288; F:356; I:583]

132 The major causes of fetal hypoxia in labour may be divided into:
(a) reversible
   (i) maternal hypotension,
   (ii) uterine overactivity;
(b) irreversible
   (i) occlusion of the umbilical cord,
   (ii) placental insufficiency.
[B:306; C:177; D:287]

133 Fetal heart rate abnormalities suggestive of fetal asphyxia can be confirmed by fetal blood sampling to determine the pH of a sample collected from the fetal scalp.
[A:358; B:307; C:173; D:289; F:359; I:588]

134 In acute hypoxia there is a failure to maintain adequate passage of O_2 from mother to fetus and a reduced excretion of CO_2 from the fetus. The build-up of CO_2 leads to a respiratory acidosis. Anaerobic glycolysis is stimulated for the production of energy and there is an accumulation of pyruvic acid and lactic acid resulting in a fall of pH.
[A:358; B:307; C:174; D:286; F:351; I:588]

135 The technique of fetal blood sampling is:
(a) visualise fetal scalp with amnioscope;
(b) clean the scalp;
(c) spray the scalp with ethyl chloride to arteriolise capillary blood;
(d) smear with silicone gel;
(e) puncture scalp with guarded blade during a contraction;
(f) collect droplet of blood into heparinised tube;
(g) measure pH.
[A:358; C:173; F:360]

136 The results of FBS may be interpreted as follows:
normal pH   7·30–7·40—repeat if further FHR change.
marginal pH   7·25–7·29—repeat in half an hour or earlier if further FHR changes occur.

fetal acidosis   7·25 or less—deliver immediately
usually by caesarean section
unless easy instrumental vaginal
delivery imminent.
[A:359; B:307; C:174; D:287; D:360; I:588]

137   Uterine contractions result in:
(a) a temporary reduction of oxygenated blood
through the intervillous space;
(b) umbilical cord compression;
(c) temporary reduction in transfer of O_2, CO_2
and metabolites.
If placental function is impaired or if contractions occur too frequently or are of too great an
intensity the cumulative reduction in transfer
may result in fetal asphyxia.
[A:353; B:306; C:166; F:351; I:581]

C   Ante natal disorders of pregnancy

Systemic diseases—cardiac

138   The main aim of ante natal management of
cardiac patients in pregnancy is the avoidance of
cardiac failure. Close cooperation between physician and obstetrician in a cardiac ante natal
clinic is desirable. Tachycardia must be avoided
and therefore such occurrences as infection,
anaemia, hypertension, obesity, arrhythmias,
must be vigorously treated. Excessive exercise
and emotional upset are also to be avoided.
[A:732; B:192; C:284; D:239; F:250; I:164]

139   A systolic murmur is a frequent occurrence in
pregnant patients. If the patient is asymptomatic with no previous history of heart
disease or rheumatic fever the murmur is almost
certainly physiological and no further action
need be taken. If the patient has a history of
heart disease or rheumatic fever or has cardio-
respiratory symptoms, a specialist cardiology
opinion is required. All diastolic murmurs require a cardiologist's assessment.
[A:780; C:281; D:239; F:219; I:159]

140   (a) The patient is asymptomatic although
clinical examination reveals heart damage.
(b) The patient is asymptomatic at rest but

normal physical exertion leads to breathlessness, fatigue and occasional palpitations.

(c) Mild exertion leads to the above symptoms but the patient is asymptomatic at rest.

(d) The patient has evidence of cardiac insufficiency at rest and is unable to take any physical exertion without considerable distress.

[A:732; C:284]

141 Termination of pregnancy is rarely indicated because of heart disease alone apart from primary pulmonary hypertension (maternal mortality rate 53 per cent) and Eisenmenger's syndrome (maternal mortality rate 27 per cent).
[A:736; B:192, C:285, I.169]

142 The two main causes of heart disease in pregnancy are rheumatic heart disease and congenital heart disease. The prevalence of rheumatic heart disease has decreased over the years and the contribution of congenital heart disease increased. Congenital heart disease now occurs as frequently as rheumatic heart disease.
[A:730; B:191; C:281; F:219; I:149]

143 The increased cardiac output and circulating blood volume will aggravate the heart condition. The worse the defect, the worse the effect.
[A:731; B:193; C:283]

144 There is some evidence to suggest that patients with heart disease have an increase in premature and small for gestational age babes. There is also an increase in the maternal mortality rate.
[A:735; C:284]

145 The indications for surgery in pregnancy do not differ from the non-pregnant state, namely failed medical treatment or the risk of developing pulmonary oedema (e.g. tight mitral stenosis) despite medical treatment.
[A:735; C:285; F:221; I:170]

146 Patients with heart disease risk developing endocarditis during labour. Antibiotics should therefore be prescribed. Regimens vary but ampicillin 500 mg 6-hourly and gentamicin

6-hourly throughout labour should be sufficient.
[A:737; B:193]

147 During the first stage of labour the cardiac patient should be nursed in Fowler's position (well propped up with legs dependent), cardiac drugs should be given intramuscularly if required. Oxygen must be immediately available as should standard resuscitative equipment.
[A:733; B:192; C:286; D:241; I:131]

148 There is no contraindication to any of the standard narcotic analgesics normally used in labour. However, morphia may well be the drug of choice in the more severe cases. Epidurals may be beneficial in patients in borderline cardiac failure as the venous return to the heart will be diminished. Care must be taken, however, to avoid hypotension.
[A:733; C:286; I:171]

149 Provided the patient is not unduly compromised or dyspnoeic, maternal effort need not be discouraged. If, after approximately 20 minutes, delivery is not imminent elective forceps delivery should be embarked upon.
[B:192; C:286; D:241; F:221; I:172]

150 Oxytocic drugs are usually given in the third stage of labour to encourage the uterus to contract, thereby reducing the risk of post partum haemorrhage (PPH). At the same time, however, 300–500 ml of blood are squeezed into the maternal circulation which may well be sufficient to precipitate cardiac failure. Oxytocic drugs should therefore be withheld in cardiac patients except those with trivial heart disease where the risk of PPH is greater than the risk of cardiac failure. In severe cases it is often wise to give morphia 10 mg intravenously and frusemide 40 mg intravenously at the onset of the third stage.
[B:192; C:287; D:241; I:172]

151 The majority of patients with artificial heart valves and mitral valve disease should be taking anticoagulants during pregnancy. Warfarin crosses the placenta and should be avoided in

the first trimester and discontinued at 32 weeks, heparin being substituted. Recently, twice daily subcutaneous heparin throughout pregnancy as a form of prophylaxis has become popular.
[A:735; B:192; C:286; I:167]

152 The only indication for inducing labour in the pregnant cardiac patient is for obstetric reasons. Await spontaneous labour if at all possible. Induction usually involves intravenous fluids and an oxytocic drug. The latter has a mild anti-diuretic effect which may be sufficient to pre-cipitate circulatory fluid overloading and cardiac failure.
[B:192; D:241; F:221; I:167]

153 Spontaneous labour usually occurs. If the pulse rate between contractions rises above 110, then digitalisation may be required. Excessive push-ing in the second stage is contraindicated and forceps delivery usually performed. Ergomet rine is avoided in the third stage for fear of over-loading the heart with a large increase in blood volume as the uterus contracts down. Antibiotic cover is mandatory.
[A:733; B:192; C:287; D:241; F:221; I:171]

Systemic diseases—anaemia

154 Erythropoiesis is increased in pregnancy as a result of increased erythropoietin stimulation by human placental lactogen.
[A:234; C:292]

155 The lowest acceptable value of haemoglobin in late pregnancy is 10·5 g although this would be unacceptable in early pregnancy.
[B:195; D:231]

156 Iron supplements in pregnancy help prevent the development of anaemia and also raise the hae-moglobin of women who are not anaemic at booking and on a good diet. The higher the hae-moglobin at term the better, as fetal require-ments are maximal in the last three months of pregnancy and blood loss at delivery may put considerable strain on the healthiest of women.
[A:313; C:293]

157 100 mg of elemental iron and 300 μg of folic acid per day is normally sufficient to prevent anaemia during pregnancy.
[A:313; C:293]

158 The two most commonly encountered anaemias of pregnancy are:
(a) iron deficiency,
(b) megaloblastic.
[A:713; B:195; I:203]

159 The common causes of anaemia in pregnancy result from:
(a) inadequate intake of iron in the diet;
(b) malabsorption;
(c) excessive blood loss—previous menor-rhagia, bleeding in pregnancy, parasite infestations;
(d) abnormal demands—multiple pregnancy, multiparity, rapidly recurring pregnancy.
[B:193; C:292; D:232; I:203]

160 Investigations of anaemia in pregnancy should include a full blood picture including examination of a blood film, serum iron, serum folate, serum B12 and serum ferritin. It may be necessary to perform haemoglobin electrophoresis or bone marrow examination, depending upon the results of the former investigations.
[A:714; B:196; C:293]

161 The effects of iron deficiency anaemia on pregnancy are:
(a) the patient is less able to withstand blood loss at delivery. In developing countries 20–30 per cent of maternal deaths are associated with severe anaemia.
(b) there is an association between acute hypertension of pregnancy and anaemia. The incidence of acute hypertension is reduced by giving iron and vitamin supplements.
(c) it predisposes to puerperal infection.
(d) there is said to be an increased incidence of premature labour and low birth weight babies.
(e) fetal distress in labour is said to be more common.
[B:193; C:295]

162 Treatment of iron deficiency anaemia in pregnancy varies with the severity of the anaemia

and duration of the pregnancy. In early pregnancy doubling the oral iron intake will raise the haemoglobin by 1 g/100 ml per month and is the method of choice. After 30 weeks' gestation, the response to oral iron is too slow and parenteral iron must be administered.
[B:197; C:293; D:233; I:204]

163 Doubling the oral iron intake of a patient who is 34 weeks pregnant and has a haemoglobin of 9·0 g/100 ml will probably not have the desired effect in time. Iron can be given as iron dextran or iron citrate—sorbitol either intramuscularly or intravenously. The total dose intravenously is preferred. The dose is calculated according to the patient's weight and the degree of anaemia.
[B:197; D:233]

164 A haemoglobin less than 9 g at 36 weeks is probably best treated by blood transfusion (one pint raises the haemoglobin by 0·7 g/100 ml). The main reason is not primarily the correction of anaemia but that further blood loss could be dangerous.
[B:197; C:293; D:234; F:214; I:208]

165 Folic acid deficiency is responsible for megaloblastic anaemia and may result from:
(a) reduced intake,
(b) diminished absorption,
(c) excess demands,
(d) diminished stores.
Anticonvulsant therapy may precipitate or aggravate folic acid deficiency and folic supplements should be prescribed for epileptics on anticonvulsant therapy.
[A:717; B:196; C:295; I:210]

166 The diagnosis of folic acid deficiency is usually made by failure of a low haemoglobin to respond to iron therapy. Serum folate levels may also be measured. A blood film is usually diagnostic.
[A:717; B:196; C:295; D:235; I:210]

167 Folic acid is necessary for the formation of nucleic acids and cell proliferation. Deficiency leads to changes in the blood film, one of which is the appearance of megaloblasts. Megaloblastic

anaemia is also sometimes caused by vitamin B12 deficiency.
[A:718; B:196; C:296; I:210]

168 It has been suggested that folic acid deficiency may result in abortion, premature labour and placental abruption. It may also be a factor in the formation of neural tube defects.
[A:718; C:296]

169 Sickle cell disease is an inherited defect in the synthesis of one of the globin chains of the hae-moglobin molecule. Adult haemoglobin con-sists of two pairs of polypeptide chains (2α and 2β chains). Both chains may be effected result-ing in homozygous sickle cell anaemia or one chain may be effected—sickle cell trait—these patients are usually asymptomatic. Homo-zygous sickle cell disease results in distorted sickle shaped red blood cells which obstruct small vessels. All black patients and those from the Mediterranean region should be screened for the disease.
[A:721; B:196; C:299; D:236; I:218]

170 In the homozygous state (haemoglobin SS) there is a 10–20 per cent mortality The condition may be considerably worsened in pregnancy. Most patients, however, are heterozygous, but hypoxic states must be avoided, especially during anaesthesia. Hypoxia may lead to sludg-ing of the blood by abnormal red cells leading to transient vascular occlusion. Dehydration and acidosis in labour may also cause this.
[A:721; B:196; C:299; D:236; I:218]

171 Regular blood transfusions are the major way of reducing complications of sickle cell disease. Infections and hypoxia should be avoided as should iron therapy as iron may be deposited in the marrow leading to haemosiderosis. Folic acid is required.
[A:721; C:299: D:237; I:218]

172 This condition occurs because of a genetic defect causing greatly reduced red cell life. The result of this haemolysis is an excess of iron in the body and iron therapy is strongly contrain-dicated. If the patient becomes severely anaemic (i.e. haemoglobin concentration below

8·0 g/100 ml), transfusion of blood may be necessary.
[A:726; B:196; C:300]

173 Neonatal thrombocytopenia occurs in 50 per cent of infants of patients with idiopathic thrombocytopenia. This is usually self-limiting. The reduced platelet count increases the risk of bleeding at delivery and lacerations or episiotomy should be avoided if possible. Platelet transfusion may be given if necessary. Steroids are normally prescribed as treatment for idiopathic thrombocytopenia in pregnancy, and splenectomy is occasionally necessary in early pregnancy.
[A:728; C:301; I:217]

174 Pregnancy does not adversely effect Hodgkin's disease and previously treated Hodgkin's disease is not a contraindication to pregnancy. Hodgkin's diagnosed in early pregnancy may be grounds for therapeutic abortion so that definitive therapy which may include radiation and administration of cytotoxic drugs can be carried out.
[A:730; C:302]

Systemic diseases—diabetes

175 There is an increased demand for a readily available source of energy during pregnancy. Human placental lactogen is an insulin antagonist and, following a glucose tolerance test or after a meal, the blood sugar level remains elevated for longer than in the non-pregnant state, thereby shifting the glucose tolerance curve to the right and facilitating placental transfer of glucose.
[A:741; C:330; D:244; F:224]

176 The incidence of diabetes mellitus in women of childbearing age is between 0·1 and 0·5 per cent. This figure rises to 1 per cent if all patients with abnormal glucose tolerance tests are included.
[A:740; B:188; C:329; D:244]

177 The fetus responds to raised levels of glucose in the maternal circulation by increasing its secretion of insulin. If the maternal levels

remain persistently high, as may be the case with a diabetic mother, then hyperplasia of the fetal islets of Langerhans will ensue.
[A:743; C:331; I:185]

178   The simplest screening test for diabetes is urine testing which is done routinely at all ante natal visits. However, approximately 60 per cent of women will have glycosuria at some stage of their pregnancy and only 2 per cent will have diabetes.
[A:741; B:188; C:330; D:246; I:183]

179   A pregnant patient presenting with glycosuria for the first time should be told to return the following week with a fasting urine specimen. If glycosuria persists, a glucose tolerance test (GTT) should be performed. Approximately 15 per cent will have abnormal glucose tolerance tests and be classified as diabetic.
[A:741; C:330; D:246; I:182]

180   A glucose tolerance test in pregnancy should be performed if the patient is potentially diabetic, i.e. has an affected sibling or a very strong family history; develops glycosuria in pregnancy on more than one occasion; has a history of a previous full term infant weighing in excess of 4·5 kg; has a history of unexplained stillbirth (particularly if post mortem analysis of the infant reveals hypertrophy of the islets of Langerhans).
[A:741; B:188; C:330; I:183]

181   To perform a GTT the patient is fasted overnight or for 12 hours. A fasting blood sugar is taken and then 50 g of glucose ingested in 200 ml of water. Blood sugars are taken every half hour for 2 hours.
[A:741; B:188; C:331; I:183]

182   The British Diabetic Association's criteria for an abnormal GTT are a fasting or 2-hour glucose level above 6·7 mmol/litre and a peak 1-hour glucose level above 10 mmol/litre.
[C:331; I:183]

183   Many women who exhibit glycosuria in pregnancy have a normal GTT because they have a lowered renal threshold for glucose.
[A:741; C:330; I:182]

184 Evidence suggests that diabetes is at least in part inherited. A history of diabetes in the mother is more significant than diabetes in the father. Approximately 7 per cent of offspring of a diabetic parent can be expected to develop the disease. This increases to 25 per cent when one or both parents develop diabetes before the age of 40.
[C:334]

185 Women delivering large babies have an approximately 50 per cent chance of developing diabetes sometime in later life.
[C:334; I:187]

186 The Kings College Hospital Classification of Diabetes in pregnancy is:
(a) diabetes diagnosed in pregnancy—gestational diabetes, accounts for approximately 15 per cent of patients.
(b) known diabetes diagnosed before pregnancy with few or no complications—the majority of patients seen.
(c) established diabetes with diabetic complications such as retinopathy or kidney disease—less than 10 per cent of patients.
[C:336]

187 The effects of diabetes on a pregnancy are:
(a) increased weight and size of the baby at birth. This in itself may lead to cephalo-pelvic disproportion and the attendant risk of difficult vaginal delivery or caesarean section.
(b) increased risk of abortion.
(c) increased risk of bacteriuria and urinary tract infection.
(d) higher incidence of hypertensive disease of pregnancy.
(e) increased incidence of vulval and vaginal candidiasis.
(f) polyhydramnios occurs in up to 50 per cent.
(g) increased risk of congenital deformities.
(h) intrauterine death, especially after 36 weeks' gestation.
(i) overall increased perinatal mortality.
[A:743; B:188; C:336; D:247; F:225; I:185]

188 There is an alteration in carbohydrate metabolism and an increasing resistance to insulin,

possibly due to the antagonistic effects of human placental lactogen (HPL). This is particularly noticeable in the last ten weeks. Diabetic lesions may become worse.
[A:742; B:189; C:335; D:247; F:225; I:190]

189 The major aim of diabetic management ante natally is to maintain the patient with as near normal blood sugar and insulin levels as possible. Levels below 8 mmol as outpatients and below 6 mmol in the last two months of pregnancy are acceptable. Maintenance should be done in conjunction with a physician with an interest in diabetes mellitus. (If you own a dog there is no point in doing the barking yourself.) Patients may need admission to hospital early in pregnancy for stabilisation. Frequent spaced doses of insulin (up to three or four times daily) are favoured in many centres. Further admission at 32 weeks is usually necessary and the patient remains in hospital for the remainder of pregnancy. Regular monitoring of blood glucose levels is necessary. Fetal welfare is closely monitored with oestriol, HPL, ultrasound measurements, daily fetal movement counts and cardiotocography. Timing of delivery depends upon the severity of the condition and the well-being of the fetus but is usual in the 37th or 38th week, although with good control the pregnancy may proceed to term and sometimes beyond. 80 per cent of diabetic patients require twice daily soluble insulin.
[A:744; B:189; C:340; D:247; F:225; I:191]

190 There is little place for oral hypoglycaemic agents in the treatment of the pregnant diabetic. Good control is more difficult and these agents cross the placenta and may cause hypoglycaemia in the neonate if not stopped 48 hours before delivery. There are no known teratogenic effects but it seems wise to avoid them in the first trimester. Occasionally a patient will become pregnant whilst on oral hypoglycaemic agents and remain well controlled, in which case this can be continued until two weeks before delivery when changeover to insulin should be instituted.
[A:746; C:341; I:193]

191 In the insulin-dependent diabetic, labour is

managed in the following way. An intravenous infusion of 5 per cent dextrose is commenced together with an insulin infusion pump containing 40 units of insulin in 40 ml of saline titrating 1–2 units of insulin per hour which may be increased or decreased according to blood sugar levels. Amniotomy and simultaneous oxytocic infusion is commenced. Hourly or 2-hourly estimations of blood glucose are made. Epidural anaesthesia is advisable to avoid maternal distress and ketosis. Caesarean section should be considered if vaginal delivery is not imminent after 8–10 hours. Other contraindications to vaginal delivery would include a previous caesarean section, primigravida over the age of 35, malpresentation, unstable lie, severe pre-eclampsia or disproportion.
[A:747; B:189; C:343; D:249; I:195]

192 The babies of diabetic mothers are usually over weight and have the appearances of having suffered a prolonged Bacchanalian orgy. They are plethoric, flabby, floppy, sleepy and often panting. They are very prone to hypoglycaemia (because of hyperinsulinaemia) and respiratory distress despite their gestational age. They often lose a considerable amount of weight in the first week of life. There is an increased incidence of congenital abnormalities (approximately 7 per cent) the most common of which are congenital heart defects but sacral agenesis, although rare, occurs more frequently in infants of diabetic mothers than in those of normal women.
[A:747; B:189; C:345; D:250; I:185]

Systemic diseases—urinary tract

193 Urinary tract infections are more common in pregnancy because there is relative urinary stasis. This is caused by a marked dilatation of the ureters and renal pelvis because of smooth muscle relaxation under the influence of pregnancy hormones. In addition, dextrorotation of the gravid uterus may compress the right ureter at the level of the pelvic brim.
[A:701; B:212; C:319; D:225; F:203; I:325]

194 In 5–10 per cent of patients, bacteria can be cultured in the urine. A midstream urine sample is

usually taken at the first attendance at an ante natal clinic as the prevalence of the development of clinical infection is as high as 30 per cent in these patients and other complications of pregnancy are more common.
[A:703, B:213; C:322; D:225; F:203; I:327]

195 Asymptomatic bacteriuria requires treatment as there is an association between it and acute pyelonephritis, anaemia and abnormalities of the renal tract. Treatment should be with a suitable antimicrobial for seven days. Recurrent urinary tract infections in pregnancy should be followed up by an IVP three months after delivery.
[A:703; B:213; C:322; D:225; F:331]

196 Ureteric colic can occur in pregnancy. Despite the hormonal effect of ureteric dilatation, stones can become lodged in the ureter. It usually occurs in the first or second trimesters of pregnancy. Diagnosis can be confirmed by emergency excretion pyelography, with the uterus shielded by a lead screen.
[A:707; C:324; I:340]

197 The causes of haematuria in pregnancy and labour are: acute urinary tract infections; trauma due to prolonged labour; forceps delivery and caesarean section. Other causes such as neoplasms, stones, sickle cell disease, placental abruption and varicose veins of the bladder should be considered.
[B:215; C:324; F:336]

198 The nephrotic syndrome is a form of chronic glomerulonephritis leading to gross proteinuria of such severity that hypoproteinaemia develops and the patient becomes markedly oedematous. Provided there is no associated hypertension the pregnancy is usually uneventful. Renal function should be assessed during pregnancy by urea and creatinine clearance estimation.
[A:708; D:227]

Systemic diseases—jaundice

199 There are three aetiological types of jaundice in pregnancy:

(a) jaundice peculiar to pregnancy—acute fatty necrosis of the liver, cholestatic jaundice, complicating severe pre-eclampsia, hyperemesis gravidarum.
(b) intercurrent jaundice—viral hepatitis, gall stones.
(c) effects of pregnancy on underlying liver disease: 40 per cent of cases are due to viral hepatitis and 20 per cent to intrahepatic cholestatic jaundice.
[A:757; B:207; C:362; F:232; I:229]

200 Acute fatty liver presents in the last trimester with jaundice, severe nausea, vomiting, abdominal pain and haematemesis usually resulting in coma and death. Lipid vacuoles are found in hepatic cells. It appears to be related to protein malnutrition and to depression of protein synthesis by certain drugs—noteably tetracyclines.
[A:758; C:363; I:234]

201 Intrahepatic cholestatic jaundice appears in the last trimester. Generalised pruritus is a feature and there may be no jaundice in mild cases. Symptoms cease two weeks after delivery but it will recur with subsequent pregnancies. The prognosis is excellent and the aetiology unknown.
[A:758; B:207; F:232; I:234]

202 It is unusual for a woman with cirrhosis to conceive and if she does spontaneous abortion is likely. Young women with juvenile cirrhosis may become pregnant and deliver normally although some patients deteriorate during each pregnancy.
[A:758]

203 Chlorpromazine, multiple exposures to halothane as well as tetracyclines may cause jaundice in pregnancy. Some drugs can cause kernicterus in the newborn—sulphonamides displace bilirubin from its binding site. Novobiocin inhibits conjugation in the liver. Phenacetin given to the mother may precipitate jaundice in an infant with glucose-6-phosphate dehydrogenase deficiency.
[C:363; F:232; I:232]

204 Hepatic function is not significantly altered in

pregnancy. Increased circulating oestrogens may result in palmar erythema and spider naevi. There is occasionally an impairment of bromsulphthalein excretion from the liver in the last trimester. Of the biochemical tests there is:
(a) slight rise in alkaline phosphatase;
(b) rise in serum cholesterol;
(c) rise in serum globulins;
(d) fall in serum albumin;
(e) fall in serum cholinesterase;
(f) transaminases are normal.
[I:229]

Systemic diseases—thyroid and adrenal

205 The free thyroxine index is the most useful investigation in investigating suspected thyroid disease.
[A:748; B:184; C:349]

206 Total T_4 and free thyroxine index should be estimated from cord blood in infants whose mothers are receiving antithyroid medication. Any abnormalities can then be recognised and corrected.
[A:750; B:185]

207 Neonatal thyrotoxicosis may result from placental transfer of long acting thyroid stimulator (LATS), an immunoglobulin produced by the mother. Once recognised, treatment should be instituted (otherwise mortality rate is 12 per cent). Treatment is only required for 3–6 weeks because the immunoglobulin will be cleared from the blood in this time.
[A:749; B:185; C:349]

208 Simple colloid goitre may be present in up to 70 per cent of pregnancies.
[A:250; C:348]

209 If a solitary nodular enlargement of the thyroid is encountered and it is hard or fixed or there are any other symptoms such as dysphagia or hoarseness, then surgical intervention is necessary in view of the probable malignant nature of the disease. If none of these features is present, give suppressive T_4 therapy. If there is no

decrease in size of the nodule again surgery should be carried out.
[C:349]

210 Hashimoto's disease. Diagnosis can be confirmed by antibody levels as it is caused by antibodies to thyroglobulin. Treatment is thyroxine to reduce the size of the gland.
[C:349]

211 Hypothyroidism is associated with infertility and rarely seen. However, if pregnancy occurs there is an increased incidence of abortion and stillbirth and mental and physical abnormality among the children. It is diagnosed by cold intolerance, decreased sweating, slow pulse and ankle jerks and a low free thyroxine index. Treatment is thyroxine until the free thyroxine index is normal.
[A:750; B:185; C:350]

212 Antithyroid drugs such as carbimazole or the thiouracils are safe if used in low doses. It is usual to give concurrent therapy of thyroxine to prevent fetal hypothyroidism. These drugs are secreted in breast milk and breastfeeding is therefore contraindicated.
[A:748; B:184; C:349]

213 Pregnancy poses a threat to patients with Addison's disease as a result of nausea and vomiting, causing sodium depletion, hypovolaemia and hypotension in the first trimester. Also labour adds a considerable strain to which the adrenal cortex may be unable to respond. Infections in pregnancy and the puerperium also add to the stress. Steroid replacement should be increased during such times.
[A:751; B:186; C:350]

214 Because of the possible increased risk of congenital abnormalities in children of mothers receiving high doses of steroids, it is advisable to reduce dosage to a minimum. ACTH should be avoided as it stimulates androgen production. In a female child some degree of virilisation could result.
[C:350; F:236]

215 Pregnancy usually aggravates the condition of

97

phaeochromocytoma. There is intermittent severe hypertension and headaches, with sweating and pallor. Cerebrovascular accidents are common with associated high mortality.
[A:751; B:186; C:351; F:236]

Systemic diseases—respiratory

216 Pulmonary tuberculosis may be diagnosed by chest X-ray, sputum culture and gastric washouts. Where tuberculosis is evident and in at-risk groups, routine ante natal chest X-ray at 14 weeks' gestation should be carried out.
[A:739; C:358; D:242; F:222; I:221]

217 Pregnancy has no effect on TB provided satisfactory medical treatment is undertaken. Flare-up in the puerperium occurs and repeat chest X-ray and sputum for culture should be carried out three months after delivery.
[A:739; C:358; D:242; F:222; I:221]

218 The management of a case of pulmonary TB in pregnancy should proceed along the following lines:
(a) explain nature of the disease;
(b) reassure the patient about the baby;
(c) warn the mother she may not be able to feed the baby or even handle it until sputum is clear and the baby vaccinated;
(d) women whose disease has been quiescent for less than two years must be warned they cannot feed the baby unless given prophylactic antituberculous therapy;
(e) infants of all women with active or inactive TB should have BCG vaccination if over 5 lbs (2·3 kg) in weight and should be segregated from the mother until Mantoux positive.
[A:739; C:358; D:242; F:222; I:222]

219 Maternal distress and hyperventilation is to be avoided in patients with a history of spontaneous pneumothorax. Epidural anaesthesia is ideal and elective forceps should be carried out in the second stage of labour.
[I:733]

220 Pneumonia causes high fever and toxicity which

may result in preterm labour or intrauterine death of the fetus. Viral pneumonia is associated with a high maternal mortality rate. Super-imposed bacterial infection must be vigorously treated.
[A:738; B:190; F:223]

221   Pregnancy has little effect on bronchial asthma. Treatment of an attack is managed in the same way as the non-pregnant state. If steroids are being administered, extra cover will be required for labour.
[A:738; B:190]

Systemic diseases—sexually transmitted diseases

222   Usually premature labour ensues and in a third of cases there is fetal death *in utero*. Congenital syphilis is characterised by snuffling due to rhinitis, rashes on the face and anogenital region, hepatosplenomegaly and marked changes in the bones, teeth and central nervous system. Treatment given before the seventh month almost invariably ensures a healthy child.
[A:752; B:170; C:361; F:234]

223   The treatment of syphilis in pregnancy is one million units of penicillin intramuscularly for 10 days. The baby should be treated with 15 000 units/kg of procaine penicillin for 10 days.
[A:752; B:170; C:361; F:234]

224   The detection of gonorrhoea in the female is difficult. A history of a purulent, yellow non-offensive vaginal or urethral discharge necess-itates urethral and cervical swabs to be taken and placed in Stuart's transport medium and thence in Thayer–Martin medium.
[A:753; B:171; C:362; D:255; F:233]

225   The treatment for gonorrhoea is 2 million units of penicillin intramuscularly.
[A:753; B:171; C:362; D:255; F:233]

226   In untreated gonorrhoea infection is transmitted to the baby during delivery causing gonococcal ophthalmia neonatorum which may cause blindness within two days unless treated. When

infection has been present in the mother, a swab from the baby's eyes should be taken for culture and prophylactic antibiotics administered.
[A:479; B:172; F:233]

227 Treatment of *Trichomonas vaginalis* infection is metronidazole 200 mg three times daily for 7 days. It should be avoided in the first trimester. The male partner should receive treatment at the same time.
[A:325; C:364; D:182]

Systemic diseases—abdominal pain

228 Painful conditions to which pregnancy predisposes are:
(a) constipation;
(b) acute hepatitis (may occur in hyperemesis gravidarum);
(c) intestinal obstruction (especially if there are adhesions from previous surgery);
(d) ovarian tumours;
(e) hiatus hernia;
(f) haematoma of rectus abdominis muscle;
(g) sickling crises.
[B:206; F:230; I:227]

229 Pain due to pregnancy in the first trimester is caused by:
(a) abortion,
(b) ectopic pregnancy,
(c) acute retention of urine,
(d) salpingitis (rare).
Pain due to pregnancy in the second trimester is caused by:
(a) acute retention of urine,
(b) red degeneration of fibroid,
(c) rupture of a pregnancy in a rudimentary horn,
(d) stretching of the round ligaments,
(e) abortion.
Pain due to pregnancy in the third trimester is caused by:
(a) placental abruption,
(b) red degeneration of fibroid,
(c) acute hypertension of pregnancy,
(d) breech presentation,
(e) labour pains,
(f) uterine rupture.
[B:206; F:230; I:227]

230 The incidental causes of pain to be considered in pregnancy include:
(a) gastroenteritis,
(b) acute appendicitis,
(c) perforation of a hollow viscus,
(d) volvulus,
(e) strangulated hernia,
(f) acute pancreatitis,
(g) renal and ureteric calculi.
[A:760; B:206; C:368; F:231; I:228]

231 The site of the pain in appendicitis is usually in the right lower quadrant but rises towards the renal angle as pregnancy advances. There are no urinary symptoms with appendicitis and the temperature seldom exceeds 38 °C. Leucocyte counts are invariably confusing but pus cells are always present in the urine in renal tract infections.
[A:760; B:206; C:370; D:226; F:230]

232 The patient complains of acute pain over one area of the uterus. She is often pyrexial. On palpation there is an acutely tender area over the uterus. A firm raised mass on the surface of the uterus may be felt but not invariably. The differential diagnosis is that of abruptio placentae.
[A:850; C:702; I:228]

Systemic diseases—viral

233 If rubella infection occurs in the first 6 weeks of pregnancy, the risk of congenital malformation is at least 50 per cent and about 30 per cent if contracted between 6 and 12 weeks.
[A:764; B:169; C:354; D:253; F:227; I:237]

234 Cataracts, deafness and cardiac abnormalities are the most common. Severe dysmaturity may also occur.
[A:764; B:169; C:354; D:253; F:227; I:237]

235 Blood is taken for an antibody titre and is repeated 2–4 weeks later. If it rises fourfold or more this is strong evidence of infection. If it is raised in the first sample and remains at approximately the same titre in the second sample, the patient is probably immune. Because

of the strong probability of the fetus being malformed, many obstetricians would recommend termination of pregnancy to an affected mother. In non-affected, non-immune patients, rubella vaccination should be offered in the puerperium.
[A:763; B:169; C:355; D:254]

236 The affects of a cytomegalovirus infection (CMV) are similar to rubella if contracted early in pregnancy. The disease in adults is usually subclinical. It may cause fetal death *in utero*.
[A:765; B:170; C:355; F:229]

237 There appears to be an association with maternal herpes infection and spontaneous abortion and the virus has been implicated as a cause of congenital anomalies. It causes infection in the newborn and thought should be given to caesarean section if active herpes infection is present.
[A:755; C:355]

238 Mumps, measles and influenza are associated with increased fetal mortality rates resulting from abortion but do not appear to cause chronic infection or congenital deformities.
[A:766; C:357]

Systemic diseases—neurological

239 There is no change in the occurrence of fits in most patients. However, medication is continued throughout pregnancy. There is an increased incidence of minor congenital defects (cleft palate and hare lip). This is probably the influence of drug therapy.
[A:772; C:358; F:235]

240 Myasthenia gravis sometimes improves, is sometimes exacerbated but often there is no change in the condition during pregnancy.
[A:773; B:181; C:359]

241 There is no indication for caesarean section on the grounds of myasthenia gravis. The myasthenic process does not effect uterine muscle and labour is usually normal. Treatment is essentially the same as in the non-pregnant

state—with anticholinesterases. 20 per cent of babies born to myasthenic mothers may have transient myasthenia.
[A:773; B:181; C:359]

242   The general opinion is that pregnancy does not aggravate the disease or influence its onset and does not constitute an indication for termination of pregnancy. However, when pregnancy occurs in the severely disabled woman termination may seem justifiable on the grounds of her relative inability to cope with the child after delivery.
[A:773; B:181; C:360]

243   Almost 75 per cent of cerebral tumours in women in the childbearing age group first present in pregnancy. The sudden appearance of convulsions and persistent vomiting should arouse suspicion.
[A:687; B:206; F:248]

244   Peripheral nerve disorders are more common in pregnancy because of an increase of mucopolysaccharides in the ground substance, fluid retention and oedema leading to compression of susceptible nerves. Carpal tunnel syndrome is particularly common. Sciatic pain is usually caused by a shift of the patient's centre of gravity.
[A:774; B:181; C:360]

Systemic diseases—bowel, skin, psychiatric

245   In patients with quiescent colitis, at the onset of pregnancy, the likelihood is that it will remain inactive throughout gestation. A recurrence is most likely in the first trimester of the puerperium. Patients with active disease at conception do less well and deterioration is likely and usually occurs in the first trimester or puerperium. Patients who develop ulcerative colitis for the first time in pregnancy have the worst prognosis and 70 per cent of patients are likely to have a severe attack placing the mother's life at risk.
[A:762; B:207; C:370]

246   There is an increased incidence of infertility in patients with Crohn's disease. However, once

pregnant there is an excellent chance of a full term live infant. The risks of abortion and stillbirth compare favourably with the normal population. There does not appear to be an increased risk of congenital abnormalities. The condition is unaffected by pregnancy and deterioration is most likely to occur in the puerperium if at all.
[A:762; C:369]

247 There is no particular mental disorder peculiar to pregnancy. Psychiatric disorders may be classified as:
(a) organic—which arise in association with physical disorders such as acute hypertension of pregnancy, severe anaemia or high fever.
(b) functional disorders—which usually have a background of psychotic disturbance before pregnancy. They fall into three groups:
(i) schizophrenia;
(ii) neuroses—hysteria, anxiety states, obsessional neurosis;
(iii) psychoses.
[B:177; F:441]

248 Unnatural sleeplessness should always arouse suspicion of psychiatric problems. Strange remarks, sudden refusal of food and on occasions unexplained pyrexia may all be forerunners to acute psychiatric upset.
[B:177; F:439]

249 The most common skin rashes resemble erythema multiforme. The rash consists of slightly raised erythematous papules which are red, itchy and oedematous. The onset may be preceded by pruritus. Herpes gestationis is a bullous eruption and much less common. It consists of itching, oedematous macules and papules which may coalesce, forming sheets. Constant scratching may produce an excoriated rash. Pruritus associated with cholestasis is common and is particularly seen in multiple pregnancy.
[A:771; C:367]

250 Ampicillin and cephalosporins. Others can be used for short periods of time but more prolonged use may cause serious side effects,

depending upon the stage of the pregnancy at which they are taken.
[B:73; C:357; F:64]

251 Heparin is safe throughout as the molecule is too large to cross into the fetal circulation. Oral anti-coagulants can be used in the second trimester but should be avoided in the last trimester because of the risks of spontaneous intracranial haemorrhage in the fetus and neonate.
[A:736; B:192; I:908]

Diseases of pregnancy—hypertension

252 Pre-eclampsia is a disease of pregnancy characterised by hypertension, generalised oedema and proteinuria. It is a disease which is generally overdiagnosed and seldom leads to true eclampsia (about 0·2 per cent).
[A:665; B:124; C:259; D:212; F:186; I:281]

253 The diastolic blood pressure must be seen to be raised above 90 mmHg over a period of time not less than 24 hours. The condition is better known as hypertensive disease of pregnancy or pregnancy induced hypertension. Systolic levels of over 140 mmHg are often implicated but are of lesser importance. An increase of systolic blood pressure greater than 30 mmHg and a diastolic blood pressure of greater than 20 mmHg over the booking clinic blood pressure are also abnormal. Fetal morbidity and mortality are raised in such cases.
[A:666; B:125; C:261; D:212; F:187; I:286]

254 The major change is of a progressive reduction in placental blood flow. The induced hypoxia leads to hyperplastic changes in both components of the trophoblast and characteristic increase in syncytial sprouting of the terminal villi, thickening of the basement membrane and swelling of the microvilli. There is decreased renal blood flow with concomitant reduction in glomerular filtration rate. There is reversible swelling of the cytoplasm of the endothelial cells of the capillaries in the glomerular tuft. Sodium retention is probably not as important as previously thought. There is generalised increase in

intracellular volume. Capillary permeability increases which, in severe cases, may lead to haemoconcentration and hypovolaemia.
[A:667; C:263; D:213]

255 The aetiology of the disease remains largely theoretical. The increased syncytial sprouting may cause maternal embolisation and thus an increase in tissue thromboplastins. This in turn could lead to disseminated intravascular coagulation. The resultant fibrinoid material accumulates in the renal glomeruli leading to decreased function. There is release of pressor substances leading to vasoconstriction and hence placental hypoxia. The initiating factors in this vicious circle are largely unknown but an alteration in maternal immune response to the fetus may be important.
[A:678; B:124; C:262; D:214; F:196]

256 A raised blood pressure before pregnancy or noted in the first half of pregnancy is likely to be due to pre-existing hypertension. Among the causes of pre-existing hypertension are:
(a) essential hypertension;
(b) renal disease (e.g. renal artery stenosis, chronic pyelonephritis);
(c) adrenal disease (e.g. phaeochromocytoma, Cushing's);
(d) collagen diseases—systemic lupus erythematosis.
(e) coarctation of aorta.
[A:696; B:193; C:260; F:200; I:311]

257 Common factors often associated with the development of hypertensive disease of pregnancy include primiparity; pre-existing hypertension or renal disease; diabetes, with cardiovascular complications; multiple pregnancy; low socioeconomic status; trophoblastic disease; obesity; elderly patients.
[B:124; C:262; F:190; I:289]

258 As well as routine examination of the cardiovascular system and abdominal palpation with a diligent search for oedema, clinical examination should include:
(a) fundoscopy,
(b) auscultation for renal bruit,
(c) palpation of femoral pulses.
[I:290]

259 Laboratory investigations in hypertensive patients should include:
   (a) 24-hour urine for creatinine clearance to check renal function and vanillyl mandelic acid (three 24-hour samples) to exclude phaeochromocytoma.
   (b) urine should be sent for microscopy and culture to rule out underlying urinary infection.
   (c) serum uric acid—levels greater than 350 nl/l are abnormal and increasing levels are an early indicator of pre-eclampsia.
   (d) serum urea and creatinine—rising levels are again significant indicators of pre-eclampsia but not as sensitive as uric acid.
   (e) platelet count and clotting screen in severe cases of pre-eclampsia.
   (f) serial plasma oestriols to assess fetoplacental function.
   [A:682; B:125; D:217; F:190; I:292]

260 The medical treatment of hypertensive disease of pregnancy depends upon the severity of the condition. In mild cases, bed rest is sufficient. In cases of persistent hypertension, medication may be of use. Sedatives are of little value as they merely serve to depress the patient and sympathetic explanation of the condition is of more value. There are three classes of hypotensives of use which may be given alone or in combination. Adrenergic blockers such as α-methyldopa are of particular value for long term use. Vasodilators such as hydrallazine are effective, particularly in more severe or acute cases. β-adrenergic blockers such as propranolol are being used increasingly. Except in very severe cases, there is no place for diuretics. Anticonvulsant therapy with diazepam has no prophylactic use (but is of considerable importance if fitting develops). There may be a place for antiepileptic drugs such as phenytoin in very severe cases.
   [A:681; B:125; C:267; D:215; F:190; I:294]

261 Delivery should be contemplated in patients with hypertensive disease:
   (a) if there is evidence of progressive placental dysfunction with fetal growth retardation. The aim of treatment is to prolong the

pregnancy until such time as the fetus is no longer at risk in an extrauterine environment.

(b) if the patient develops eclampsia.

(c) if there is rapid deterioration in the patient's condition (e.g. uncontrolled hypertension, cerebral haemorrhage, hepatic subcapsular haemorrhage).

[A:683; B:125; C:269; D:216; F:295]

262　The management of this patient entails admission to hospital and bed rest. Ultrasonic examination for the first time is of little value at this late stage but may be helpful if previous scans have been performed. Oestriol estimations are of limited value at this stage unless performed serially. Cardiotocography is of use. If the blood pressure settles the patient may return home. If it remains elevated, then there may be an indication for induction, especially if proteinuria develops.

[A:682; B:125; C:268; D:216; F:190; I:295]

263　If the diastolic blood pressure exceeds 110 mmHg parenteral antihypertensive therapy is indicated. The drug of choice is hydrallazine intramuscularly or intravenously. A commonly used regimen is 10 mg hydrallazine given slowly intravenously followed by 40 mg in 500 ml dextrose 5 per cent titrating 2–20 mg of hydrallazine per hour according to the blood pressure. Alternatively 5–10 mg of hydrallazine may be given intravenously as a bolus repeatedly in order to keep the blood pressure below 110 mmHg.

[A:690; F:192; I:298]

264　The signs of impending eclampsia are:

(a) persistent headache,

(b) raised blood pressure and proteinuria,

(c) generalised oedema,

(d) visual disturbance—flashing lights, spots,

(e) hyperreflexia and restlessness,

(f) oliguria.

(g) epigastric pain

[A:684; B:128; C:270; D:218; F:193; I:297]

265　The management of a patient with eclampsia will entail maintenance of airway, control of fits and hypertension, monitoring of urine output by means of indwelling catheter and fluid replacement as indicated by central venous

pressure monitoring. Fetal monitoring should be instituted and coagulation studies performed. Coagulation defects should be corrected if present. Following control of the hypertension and fits, delivery of the infant will be required—this will usually entail caesarean section unless vaginal delivery is imminent.
[A:684; B:128; C:270; D:219; F:194; I:298]

266 Drugs commonly used to control eclamptic fits include:
   (a) diazepam as a bolus (10 mg i.v.) and titrated as a solution of 40 mg in 500 ml dextrose 5 per cent;
   (b) chlormethiazole 0·8 per cent solution titrated until the patient is sleepy;
   (c) magnesium sulphate 20 per cent solution—favoured in the USA. 4 g i.v. are given over 5 minutes and 5 g into each buttock i.m. followed by 5 g i m 4-hourly until 24 hours after delivery.
[A:688; B:128; C:271; D:219; F:194; I:198]

Diseases of pregnancy—rhesus disease

267 The rhesus factor is a complex antigen consisting of three pairs of genes (CDE) occupying a specific locus on the chromosome. Only the D pair are of importance in rhesus isoimmunisation.
[A:961; C:307; D:258; F:447; I:980]

268 Rhesus isoimmunisation occurs by the passage of incompatible fetal red cells into the maternal circulation. This usually occurs during the third stage of labour but can occur after abortion, ectopic pregnancy, external cephalic version, amniocentesis, ante partum haemorrhage or spontaneously.
[C:308; D:258; F:448; I:981]

269 Depending upon the severity of the disease, the fetus may suffer from:
   (a) haemolytic anaemia. In this case, anaemia is present at birth—between 14 g and 18 g per 100 ml. There may be jaundice some days after delivery. Blood transfusion may be necessary.
   (b) haemolytic jaundice. There is marked

anaemia and the bilirubin is raised at birth. The liver and spleen are enlarged. Exchange transfusion is necessary to prevent kernicterus and irreversible brain damage.

(c) hydrops fetalis. Anaemia is so severe *in utero* that the fetus goes into heart failure and dies. There is characteristic oedema, ascites and hepatosplenomegaly.

[A:966; C:310; D:262; F:449; I:986]

270   Most ABO antibodies are of the IgM type (macroimmunoglobulins) and do not cross the placental barrier. Rhesus antibodies are a mixture of IgM and IgG immunoglobulins, the latter crossing the placental barrier and causing red cell destruction in the rhesus-positive fetus.
[B:137; C:307; F:448; I:981]

271   In pregnancy, fetal cells enter the maternal circulation in very small numbers. If the ABO group of the fetus is incompatible with the mother, the cells will be destroyed before an allergic response leading to rhesus antibody formation can occur.
[B:137; C:307; F:448; I:981]

272   Yes. If the father's genotype is Dd (i.e. he is heterozygous), his blood group will be represented as rhesus-positive because D is dominant. However, a rhesus-negative woman (dd) and a heterozygous rhesus-positive man (Dd) have an even chance of producing a rhesus-negative child.
[B:137; I:982]

273   Blood is examined for antibodies at the first antenatal clinic attendance and subsequently at 28 weeks and 36 weeks. These tests will be carried out more frequently if antibodies are detected.
[B:137; C:313; I:251; F:450; I:989]

274   Amniocentesis is performed. The level of bilirubin in the liquor, as measured by spectrophotometry, correlates directly with the amount of fetal red cell destruction. The same is not true for maternal antibody titres.
[A:966; B:138; C:313; D:259; I:990]

275   Maternal blood is taken for the Kleihauer elution

test. In this, the blood is mixed with a specific elutant which causes haemolysis of adult red cells but not of fetal cells. An accurate assessment of fetal transfusion of the mother can be made. Fetal blood is taken from the placenta for an assessment of haemoglobin, ABO and rhesus grouping, bilirubin concentration and the direct Coombs test.
[A:971; B:138; D:262; F:450; I:1000]

276 A rhesus-negative woman who gives birth to a rhesus-positive baby, and in whom there is evidence of transfusion of fetal red cells (Kleihauer test), is given an intramuscular injection of anti-D gammaglobulin. This material 'mops up' any circulating fetal red cells and prevents the patient from forming her own antibodies. It must be given within 72 hours of the transfusion and only to women who have no demonstrable antibodies. In many centres, the Kleihauer test is no longer performed and anti-D given to all rhesus-negative mothers at the termination of their pregnancy, be it full term or before.
[A:963; B:139; C:310; D:261; F:451; I:1004]

Diseases of pregnancy—hyperemesis gravidarum

277 Hyperemesis is a progression of morning sickness to a degree where vomiting occurs throughout the day, even if no food is taken.
[A:322; B:205; C:368; D:178; I:247]

278 Hyperemesis gravidarum leads to dehydration, electrolyte disturbance and ketosis. When ketonuria is present, hospital admission is necessary as the vomiting is having a serious metabolic effect. If untreated, CNS signs (polyneuritis), jaundice and oliguria may result, the patient eventually developing Wernicke's encephalopathy.
[B:205; D:178; I:248]

279 Treatment of a case of severe vomiting in pregnancy requires exclusion of causes not associated with the pregnancy such as urinary tract infection, hiatus hernia etc. It is also essential to rehydrate the patient. Electrolyte balance must first be checked and then an intravenous infusion of 10 per cent dextrose commenced.

Nothing is given by mouth. Pulse and blood pressure must be checked repeatedly and the urine tested for ketones, protein and sugar on each occasion that it is voided. Antiemetics may be of some use but in the acute phase the oral route is not favoured.
[B:205; D:178; I:250]

280   Charlotte Bronte died from hyperemesis gravidarum.

Bleeding in pregnancy

281   An ante partum haemorrhage may be defined as any bleeding from the birth canal after the 28th week of pregnancy and before the birth of the baby.
[B:116; C:248; D:201; F:157; I:420]

282   The causes of ante partum haemorrhage are:
(a) vulval—trauma, varicosities;
(b) vaginal—infection, trauma;
(c) cervical—polyps, carcinoma, trauma;
(d) uterine—placenta praevia, placental abruption and other placental conditions.
In at least 30 per cent of all cases there will be no obvious cause for the bleeding but it must be presumed to be placental in the absence of any other evidence.
[B:116; C:248; D:203; F:157; I:421]

283   In this condition, which usually occurs in the third trimester, there is partial or total separation of the placenta with blood loss. This loss may vary from minimal to life endangering. The condition is nearly always accompanied by pain and an accompanying area of tenderness over the uterus.
[A:495; B:116; C:252; D:209; F:158; I:455]

284   Increasing parity is the most important. In one-fifth of cases there may be associated pre-eclampsia but this often develops after the haemorrhage possibly as a result of disseminated intravascular coagulation. The condition is more common in lower socioeconomic groups but no definite dietary deficiency has been satisfactorily demonstrated.
[A:496; B:117; C:251; D:207; F:158; I:456]

285   Concealed, revealed and mixed. The blood loss
       may be entircly retroplacental (concealed), or
       due to separation of the placental edge and
       usually totally vaginal in presentation (re-
       vealed); or a combination of the two (mixed).
       The latter is the most common but remember the
       revealed element may be only a small fraction of
       the total loss. Therefore never assess blood loss
       visually in cases of placental abruption.

286   Where there is no circulatory collapse and no
       evidence of immediate fetal distress, the patient
       with a mild placental abruption is confined to
       bed for at least two days after the cessation of
       bleeding. Routine serial screening measures
       (e.g. oestriol estimations and ultrasound
       scanning) are carried out for the remainder of
       the pregnancy and the labour is induced at term
       or before.
       [A:498; B:117; C:252; D:209; F:162; I:470]

287   In the case of severe placental abruption, the
       patient is in a state of cardiovascular shock and
       immediate resuscitative measures must be
       taken. A central venous pressure line is desir-
       able and bladder catheterisation necessary to
       monitor renal function. The patient may have an
       acutely tender uterus and termination of the
       pregnancy must be carried out immediately. If
       the fetus is still alive and the gestational age
       exceeds 32 weeks, emergency caesarean section
       is usually performed but there is a real danger of
       a consumptive coagulopathy and uncontrollable
       haemorrhage. If the fetus is dead, rupture of the
       membranes with simultaneous oxytocic
       infusion is undertaken. The most important
       measure is rapid and complete replacement of
       lost blood which can only effectively be judged
       by using central venous pressure monitoring.
       [A:501; B:118; C:252; D:210; F:163; I:476]

288   Placenta praevia occurs when the placenta is
       wholly or partly situated in the lower segment of
       the uterus. Four degrees are described:
       (a) first degree—the placenta lies partly in the
           lower segment but does not encroach upon
           the internal os.

(b) second degree—the placental edge extends up to the internal os but does not cover it.
(c) third degree—the placenta covers the internal os when closed but only partially when dilated.
(d) fourth degree—the placenta lies centrally over the internal os.

First and second degree are known as minor placenta praevia and third and fourth as major placenta praevia.
[A:508; B:119; C:253; D:203; F:116; I:423]

289 The typical presentation of a patient with placenta praevia is that of small, recurrent painless bleeds. Subsequent bleeding may become increasingly profuse and life endangering. There is no significant abdominal pain or tenderness. In the majority of cases the bleeding occurs after 28 weeks. The presenting part is almost always high and unstable.
[A:510; B:120; C:249; D:204; F:168; I:424]

290 Placental localisation may be performed by:
(a) Radiology may be helpful in that soft tissue masses such as the placenta can be visualised but it is very inaccurate. Percutaneous femoral angiography is the most accurate form of placentography but it is highly invasive, has an unacceptable morbidity and exposes the fetus to unnecessary radiation.
(b) Isotope scanning using radium or technetium is useful and involves very little radiation to the fetus. The placenta concentrates the radioisotope because of the large pool of blood contained within it.
(c) Thermography—this has proved disappointing and inaccurate.
(d) Ultrasound—a B scan of the uterus is the most acceptable method now in use. It is harmless to mother and fetus and has a high degree of accuracy in experienced hands.
(e) Vaginal examination—this can *only* be carried out under general anaesthesia in a theatre prepared to proceed immediately to caesarean section. The procedure may be undertaken in patients over 38 weeks pregnant who present with painless bleeding.
[A:511; B:120; C:250; D:202; F:169; I:434]

291 The management of mild vaginal bleeding in the third trimester is as follows.
(a) The patient must be admitted to hospital.
(b) A careful history is taken especially with reference to pain.
(c) General examination and gentle palpation of the abdomen is performed to assess uterine tone, tenderness, the position of the fetus. The fetal heart rate is counted. Under no circumstances is a vaginal examination performed.
(d) Blood is taken for grouping and cross-matching.
(e) Intravenous infusion is commenced.
(f) Continuous fetal heart monitoring should be started wherever possible.
(g) Nursing observations (e.g. pulse, blood pressure, etc.) are continued for at least a few hours on a half hourly basis or more frequently.
(h) If there is no further bleeding, placental localisation should be performed, preferably by ultrasound. There being no evidence of placenta praevia, a speculum examination of the vagina and cervix may then be carried out.
[A:513; B:122; C:253; D:205; F:170; I:429]

292 The patient must be treated conservatively in hospital. Cross-matched blood must be available at all times. The aim is to maintain the pregnancy until the fetus is mature. Emergency caesarean section may be necessary if heavy bleeding develops but elective section is otherwise carried out in the 37th or 38th week in all major degrees of placenta praevia.

In first degree placenta praevia, the head may engage in the pelvis and under these circumstances examination under anaesthesia (with full preparation for caesarean section) may be undertaken. If no placenta is felt through the vaginal fornices rupture of the membranes is carried out.
[A:513; B:122; C:253; D:205; F:170; I:429]

293 At this late stage of pregnancy, delivery is advisable. The patient is prepared for caesarean section. Under general anaesthesia, the patient is placed in the lithotomy position and a very careful vaginal examination made. A finger is

not introduced through the cervix until each of the four fornices is examined and fetal head felt. If a soft mass is felt to be intervening this is assumed to be placenta, and caesarean section is carried out immediately. If no placenta is felt, the membranes are ruptured and synthetic oxytocic infusion commenced. The patient is allowed to labour normally. It must be stressed that this examination should only ever be undertaken in a theatre fully prepared for caesarean section with all the necessary staff scrubbed up and ready to proceed immediately.
[A:513; B:122; C:253; D:206; F:170; I:429]

294   Other placental causes of ante partum haemorrhage include rupture of a marginal vein of the placenta, circumvallate placenta and vasa praevia.
[B:122; F:156; I:428]

295   On rare occasions the umbilical cord is attached to the placental bed by a leash of vessels rather than centrally inserted. If these vessels cross the internal cervical os, they can be traumatised when membranes are ruptured. Fetal bleeding results which quickly results in exsanguination of the fetus. Delivery must be prompt by caesarean section but very often the fetus succumbs.
[A:574; B:122; I:428]

296   The Apt test may be used to distinguish between fetal and maternal blood. A sample of the blood is taken from the vagina and sodium hydroxide added. Maternal haemoglobin is denatured by the alkali and turns yellow/brown but fetal haemoglobin is relatively resistant to denaturation.
[A:575; B:122; I:429]

Liquor amnii

297   The amniotic fluid protects the developing fetus from external forces; it allows free movement of the limbs and equal growth of the fetus in all directions; it enables essential functions such as swallowing, fetal 'breathing', and urination; it protects the fetus from infection.
[A:206; B:130]

298   300 ml, 1000 ml, and 600 ml respectively.
       [A:206; B:130; C:400; D:269]

299   Polyhydramnios is an excessive accumulation of
       liquor in excess of 2000 ml at term.
       [A:578; B:130; C:401; D:269; F:173; I:377]

300   The common causes of polyhydramnios are
       multiple pregnancy (more common in uniovular
       twins); pregnancy associated with maternal dia-
       betes; conditions affecting the swallowing
       mechanism such as anencephaly; tracheo-
       oesophageal fistula; congenital abnormalities—
       particularly achondroplasia; idiopathic.
       [A:578; B:131; C:402; D:269; F:173; I:377]

301   Radiology of the abdomen to exclude fetal
       abnormality and multiple pregnancy and a glu-
       cose tolerance test are usually performed. If the
       uterus is particularly tense, slow release of
       liquor via a fine polythene catheter can be
       carried out but this carries the risk of infection
       and premature membrane rupture and usually
       has a very temporary effect. At birth a tube must
       be passed into the baby's stomach to exclude
       oesophagial atresia.
       [A:580; B:130; C:403; F:175; I:377]

302   Oligohydramnios may be defined as a volume of
       amniotic fluid less than 200 ml. In 50 per cent of
       patients no obvious abnormality will be found in
       such patients. However, in other cases, it may
       signify either placental failure and intrauterine
       growth retardation or fetal malformation. The
       usual fetal malformation is renal agenesis or ob-
       struction of the lower urinary tract preventing
       urination by the fetus.
       [A:581; B:131; D:270]

D   Normal labour

Physiology

303   During labour a number of physiological
       changes occur:
       (a) considerable expenditure of energy (result-
           ing in ketoacidosis if not prevented). The
           increased energy production results in in-
           creased heat production and sweating
           occurs.

(b) the cardiac output rises as a result of increased heart rate. The blood pressure also rises.

(c) body temperature rises up to 37·8 °C but may exceed this if ketosis develops.

(d) the motility of the intestinal tract is reduced and gastric emptying delayed.

[B:231; D:105]

304 During labour the fetal head may undergo caput formation and moulding. It undergoes a greater or lesser degree of hypoxia depending on fetal and placental reserves. It is susceptible to changes in maternal circulation such as acidosis or low blood sugar levels.
[B:231]

305 The uterus is made up of three muscle layers: an important middle spiral layer and rather poorly developed inner circular and outer longitudinal layers. The amount of muscle tissue gradually diminishes as the cervix is approached. The cervix contains only 10 per cent muscle tissue; the rest is made up of fibrous and connective tissue.
[B:19; C:107]

306 Braxton Hicks contractions are painless physiological contractions of the uterus mainly observed in the third trimester. They may aid in thinning the lower segment.
[A:223; B:4; C:181; D:100; F:36]

307 Factors that may be involved in the initiation of labour are: distension of the uterus; change in the 'protective' action of progesterone; oxytocin release by the fetal pituitary; corticosteroid secretion by the fetal adrenal; position of the presenting part in relationship to the cervix.
[A:369; C:181]

308 At the junction of the fallopian tube and uterus on each side is a 'pacemaker', one side being dominant. The uterine contractions originate from this pacemaker and spread inwards and downwards at a rate of 2 cm per second to involve the entire uterus.
[B:227; C:181; I:565]

309   A coordinate uterine contraction simultane-
       ously thins and draws up the lower uterine seg-
       ment around the presenting part and also causes
       descent of the presenting part.
       [A:377; B:229; C:181]

310   The uterus contracts throughout pregnancy and
       the contractions are of two basic types depend-
       ing upon whether oestrogen or progesterone is
       predominant.
       (a) A waves—low amplitude (0·2 mmHg in-
            trauterine pressure) high frequency contrac-
            tions under the influence of oestrogen;
       (b) B waves—increased amplitude but lower
            frequency contractions as a result of in-
            creased progesterone secretion.
       For the first 30 weeks of pregnancy A waves
       occur on average once a minute while B waves
       occur approximately once per hour. In the last 10
       weeks of pregnancy B waves increase in fre-
       quency and amplitude and are one of the main
       factors causing cervical 'ripening'.
       [A:377; C:109]

311   Effacement of the cervix results in shortening of
       the cervical canal until it is replaced by a thin
       circular orifice.
       [A:382; B:226]

312   The lower segment of the uterus is that part of
       the uterus between the internal os of the cervix
       and the line of reflection of the uterine perito-
       neum onto the bladder. The amount of muscle
       diminishes throughout pregnancy and is re-
       placed by fibrous tissue. As a consequence it
       becomes stretched in late pregnancy as it is
       drawn up around the presenting part.
       [A:378; B:226; I:421]

313   Bandl's ring is the physiological ring between
       the thick upper segment and thin lower seg-
       ment.
       [A:380; B:226; I:616]

314   As the uterus contracts the upper segment
       thickens and changes from a globular to longi-
       tudinal shape. This has the effect of
       straightening the fetal spine so that the fundus
       may press the presenting part into the pelvis,

and as the uterus lengthens so the lower segment is pulled up and stretched over the lower pole of the fetus. In obstructed labour the lower segment becomes extremely thin and Bandl's ring may become prominent and palpable. It is then known as the pathological retraction ring of Bandl.
[A:380; B:227]

315 It is not clearly understood what causes the pain of uterine contractions because the intensity of contractions after delivery are of equal intensity as those in labour but are relatively painless. It may in part be due to ischaemia, the pain from ischaemic muscle at the fundus being referred along T12 and experienced as central abdominal pain. Excessive stretching of the lower segment as occurs in malpresentation results in stimulation of the paracervical nerve plexus resulting in referred pain into the back—hence backache.
[F:70; D:102]

316 The operculum is a mucus plug, formed under progestogenic influence, situated in the endocervical canal. It prevents entry of bacteria into the uterine cavity to some extent. It is lost at the commencement of labour or before.
[B:228]

317 The normal intrauterine resting pressure in pregnancy is approximately 5 mmHg. During the height of a contraction this might rise to 60–100 mmHg.
[A:377; B:227; C:181]

Pain relief

318 Psychoprophylaxis is a technique designed to prepare the mother and allay her fears of labour. It is based on the Pavlovian theory of conditioned automatic reflex actions. The patient is taught a set of daily physical exercises, the skill of relaxation and three depths of conscious controlled breathing, a focus of activity to further raise her pain threshold.
[B:238; D:72; I:616]

319 Narcotic drugs commonly used in labour include:

(a) pethidine (meperidine),
(b) omnopon,
(c) pentazocine,
(d) morphine.
[B:239; D:153; F:364; I:591]

320 The advantages of narcotic analgesia in labour
     are:
     (a) the ease of administration,
     (b) the rapidity of action,
     (e) easily reversible,
     (d) low incidence of serious side effects.
     [B:239; D:153; I:592]

321 The major side effect of narcotic drugs that are
     used in labour is that they depress the respira-
     tory centres of mother and baby. The effect on
     the baby can be reversed by naloxone given in-
     tramuscularly.
     [A:438, B:239, I:592]

322 The main inhalational analgesics available are:
     (a) nitrous oxide/oxygen. This mixture is very
         useful as it is non-toxic, rapidly acting, has
         no affect on the fetus, very few side effects
         and is self-administered.
     (b) penthrane (methoxyfluorane). This agent
         has a rather sweet, unpalatable smell. It is
         equally effective as nitrous oxide but its
         popularity is declining.
     (c) trilene (trichlorethylene). This is seldom
         used nowadays. It has a cumulative effect
         on the mother and may depress the baby.
         Cardiac arrhythmias have been reported.
     [A:439; B:240; D:153; F:365; I:595]

323 Epidural analgesia is a method of pain relief pro-
     viding complete analgesia from the level of T10
     down to and including the perineum. It is
     accomplished by the injection of local anaesthe-
     tic (e.g. Bupivicaine) into the peridural space
     through a fine plastic catheter passed into the
     space via a Tuohy needle inserted between a
     lumbar vertebral space or the sacral hiatus.
     [A:450; B:243; C:480; F:364; I:600]

324 The major complications of epidural anaesthesia
     are:
     (a) puncture of the dura leading to excessive

leakage of cerebrospinal fluid resulting in severe headaches.
(b) inadvertant spinal anaesthesia leading to respiratory arrest.
(c) hypotension—this is common and often a desired effect (e.g. in the severe pre-eclamptic patient) but may lead to placental underperfusion and fetal distress.
(d) permanent nerve injury—this is excessively rare.
(e) loss of bladder function which may occur up to 24 hours after delivery.
[A:451; B:243; C:481; F:364; I:601]

325 Before an epidural cannula is inserted, an intravenous infusion must be commenced. In the advent of a hypotensive crisis, the patient should be nursed in a left lateral position and the intravenous infusion rate rapidly increased.
[A:452]

326 The main contraindications to epidural anaesthesia are: patient refusal, recent ante partum haemorrhage, sepsis at the site of proposed injection, bleeding problems, central nervous system disease and sensitivity to the drugs used. Breech presentation is no longer considered a contraindication and many authorities would consider it a positive help in cases of footling presentation. Cephalopelvic disproportion cannot be proven until a patient is allowed to go into labour and is not a contraindication to epidural anaesthesia.
[A:452; B:244; I:601]

327 The major complications of general anaesthesia in labour are:
(a) inhalation of stomach contents—Mendelson's syndrome;
(b) hypoxia resulting from a failure to intubate;
(c) cardiac arrest.
[A:440; B:246; F:367]

328 Mendelson's syndrome is a condition characterised by cyanosis and collapse of the patient caused by acute bronchospasm and gross impairment of pulmonary function. It is often lethal. It arises following inhalation of gastric contents causing a chemical pneumonitis. It is

believed that the low pH of gastric fluid leads to the pneumonitis.
[A:441; B:247; C:479; F:368]

329   Patients are not allowed to take anything by mouth except sips of water. Magnesium trisilicate mixture or other antacids are administered orally every 2 hours in an effort to raise the pH. If general anaesthesia is needed, a cuffed endotracheal tube must be used and suction must always be available.
[A:441; B:247; C:479; F:368]

330   Analgesia for forceps delivery may be provided by:
(a)   perineal infiltration with local anaesthetic (1 per cent lignocaine);
(b)   pudendal block;
(c)   epidural anaesthesia;
(d)   spinal anaesthesia (an anaesthetic injected directly intrathecally into the cerebrospinal fluid);
(e)   general anaesthesia.
[D:157; F:367]

331   A pudendal block is carried out transvaginally by injecting 10 ml of 1 per cent lignocaine through a pudendal needle 0·5 cm below the ischial spines. It is satisfactory for mid- and low-cavity forceps and ventouse extraction—it may not, however, be sufficient for rotational forceps when epidural, spinal or general anaesthesia should be considered.
[A:445; B:245; D:155; F:366; I:634]

Diagnosis and first stage

332   The three stages of labour are:
1st stage—from the onset of labour to full dilatation of the cervix.
2nd stage—from full dilatation to delivery of the baby.
3rd stage—from delivery of the baby to expulsion of the placenta and membranes.
[A:375; B:228; D:113; F:69]

333   Labour is defined as the process by which the fetus, placenta and membranes are expelled

through the birth canal. Normal labour is described as one in which the fetus is born at term and presents by the vertex, the process being completed spontaneously within 24 hours with no complications arising.
[B:226; D:112]

334 By the presence of rhythmical contractions occurring at least every 5 minutes accompanied by either a show, rupture of the membranes or evidence of *progressive* cervical dilatation. As the diagnosis is initially made by the patient, it is not surprising that she is often wrong. A patient who has strong regular contractions but has no evidence of cervical dilatation or membrane rupture is *not* in labour and under no circumstances should be admitted to the labour ward.
[B:228; D:112; F:70]

335 All patients who are suspected of being in labour must be examined vaginally on admission, and the state and dilatation of the cervix assessed. This examination should be repeated one or two hours later (but no later) and only if there has been a change in dilatation or descent of the presenting part, can progress be said to have been made.
[A:406]

336 Observation of the woman in labour should include assessment of:
(a) uterine contractions,
(b) dilatation of the cervix,
(c) descent of the presenting part,
(d) discharge from the vagina,
(e) fetal condition,
(f) maternal condition and the recognition of complications that may arise.
[B:233; D:120; F:115]

337 During vaginal examination in labour, assessment is made of:
(a) state of the vagina;
(b) dilatation and effacement of the cervix;
(c) presence or absence of forewaters;
(d) character of the liquor (presence or absence of meconium or blood);
(e) position of the presenting part;
(f) level of the presenting part (station).
[A:406; B:232; D:121]

338　The station of the presenting part is the level of the presenting part in relation to the ischial spines on vaginal examination.
[A:407; B:234; D:122]

339　Information regarding the descent of the fetal head can be obtained by two methods:
(a) abdominal palpation—where the level of the fetal head is expressed in terms of fifths of the fetal head still palpable above the pelvic brim. Five fifths is equivalent to a floating head and zero fifths to one that is deeply engaged.
(b) vaginal examination—with reference to the station of the presenting part.
[A:407; B:232; D:123; I:578]

340　Normal labour is characterised by the passage of pale clear liquor. If the membranes have been ruptured for longer than 24 hours the liquor may become offensive and the fetus and birth canal may become infected. The presence of fresh meconium in the liquor suggests fetal distress except in cases of breech presentation. Blood in the liquor may signify placental separation or uterine rupture. Golden liquor is seen in some cases where the fetus is suffering from rhesus haemolytic disease.
[B:132; F:351]

341　A partogram is a visual record of progress in labour, usually represented as a graph with hours of labour on one axis and cervical dilatation on the other.
[B:229; C:415; D:124; F:116; I:578]

342　The first stage of labour can be divided into
(a) latent phase,
(b) active phase.
[A:387; B:229; C:186; D:113]

343　The latent phase of labour is the stage of labour (lasting about 5–8 hours in primigravid patients) in which there is slow progressive dilatation of the cervix with descent of the presenting part.
[A:387; B:229; C:186; D:113]

344　The active phase of labour begins at a point in time when the rate of dilatation changes. For practical purposes it may be defined as being

when the cervix is 3 cm dilated and 100 per cent effaced. In the active phase the cervix dilates at a maximum of 3 cm per hour in primigravidae and almost 6 cm per hour in multigravidae. The average length of the active phase in primigravidae is 5 hours (±3·5 hours) and in the multigravidae, the average length of the active phase is 2 hours (±1·5 hours).
[A:387; B:229; C:186; D:114]

345 The most common position at the start of labour is left occipitotransverse (LOT).
[A:395; B:248; C:187; D:113; F:90]

346 The diameter of the fetal skull presented when the head is flexed is the suboccipitobregmatic. It is approximately 9·5 cm at full term.
[B:26; D:92]

347 Asynclitism results when the head engages through the pelvic brim with the sagittal suture in the transverse diameter. If the suture should lie nearer the sacral promontory or symphysis pubis then asynclitism (anterior or posterior) exists, resulting in one or other of the parietal bones being predominant on vaginal examination.
[A:396; B:251; D:108]

348 It is an oedematous swelling of the fetal scalp caused by pressure of the fetal head on a partially dilated cervix.
[A:403; B:26; D:94; F:74]

349 Moulding is a change in the shape of the fetal skull that occurs during its passage through the pelvis. The parietal bones slip under each other and the frontal and occipital bones slip under the parietal bones.
[A:403; B:27; D:94; F:75]

Second stage of labour

350 The objectives of management of the second stage of labour are:

(a) to ensure a healthy undamaged live child;
(b) to preserve the muscles of the perineum;
(c) to prevent infection of the genital tract.
[D:124]

351   The onset of the second stage of labour may be
      heralded by:
      (a) increase in intensity of contractions;
      (b) an urge to bear down or defaecate;
      (c) dilatation of the anus;
      (d) vomiting or nausea;
      (e) distension of the perineum.
      [A:414; B:230; D:124]

352   The average length of the second stage of labour
      is 40 minutes for the primigravidae and 20
      minutes for the multigravidae. Delivery should
      not be attempted merely because a set time has
      elapsed. Provided the fetal condition is
      satisfactory and progressive descent of the
      presenting part is taking place, no intervention is
      needed. Not infrequently, a normal second stage
      will last well over an hour in primigravid
      patients.
      [B:230; D:116]

353   During the second stage the following should be
      noted:
      (a) the patient should be nursed on her side until
           the head reaches the perineum, then turned
           onto her back;
      (b) vaginal discharge should be noted for
           meconium and blood in particular;
      (c) the maternal pulse and BP should be checked
           every 15 minutes;
      (d) the bladder must be empty, catheterised if
           necessary;
      (e) parenteral analgesics should not be given;
      (f) instruct and encourage the patient to bear
           down;
      (g) never leave the patient unattended;
      (h) record the fetal heart every 5 minutes and
           during and after every contraction unless
           continuous monitoring is in progress.
      [A:414; B:236; F:120; D:124; I:579]

354   (a) The dorsal position. The patient lies on her
           back in a semi-sitting position, with knees
           flexed and widely apart. During pushing she
           draws her knees up to the abdomen. It is the

most common position adopted in labour suites in the UK.

(b) The left lateral position. This position requires an assistant to support the right leg. The advantage is excellent head control by the accoucheur with better protection of the perineum. It is far from natural for the patient and has lost favour in recent years.

(c) The lithotomy position. This is almost mandatory for instrumental deliveries but has definite disadvantages for the patient who may feel restrained by the position. The patient is also at greater risk if inhalation of gastric contents occurs.

(d) The squatting position. This is probably the most natural position to adopt and easiest for the patient, but control of the delivery of the head is difficult for the accoucheur.

[B:253; D:126]

355 The movements that the fetus undergoes to negotiate the birth canal when the head is presenting and is fully flexed may be summarised as follows: engagement, flexion, internal rotation, descent, extension of the head, birth of the head, restitution, external rotation.
[A:396; B:249; D:115]

356 Crowning is the point at which the leading part of the head distends the perineum. The head is fully flexed and, for birth to occur extension of the head follows.
[B:4; D:116]

357 Restitution is the untwisting of the head on the neck caused previously by internal rotation of the head to the occiput anterior position. Internal rotation of the shoulders to the anteroposterior position causes further external rotation of the head.
[A:401; B:253; D:116]

358 Following the birth of the head, a finger is placed past the occiput to ascertain whether the cord is around the neck. Excess mucus is removed from the baby's mouth and nose. If there is meconium present, then aspiration may be necessary.
[B:260; D:127; F:120]

359 When nuchal entanglement of the cord is found

on delivery of the baby's head, if the cord is loose, it may be drawn over the baby's head or if it is tight, it is divided between two clamps.
[A:420; B:260]

Third stage of labour

360 (a) The placenta presents at the vulva with the fetal surface showing. The membranes follow and then retroplacental clot (Schultze).
(b) The placenta slides out edge first, the maternal surface being seen first. Bleeding often occurs prior to the delivery of the placenta (Matthews, Duncan).
[A:389; C:192]

361 There are two ways of managing the third stage of labour:
(a) physiologically,
(b) actively.
[B:264; D:128; F:123]

362 Physiological management of the third stage allows time for the natural separation of the placenta. This usually takes 10–15 minutes to occur. Oxytocic drugs are not administered.
[A:423; D:130; I:750]

363 Placental separation may be indicated by lengthening of the cord with a rise in the uterine fundus. There is often a small show of blood. The signs represent the placenta being expelled into the vagina. Separation of the placenta occurs as a result of a marked reduction in the surface area of the uterus after delivery of the baby, uterine contractions and retroplacental bleeding.
[A:423; B:264; D:130; F:123; I:751]

364 The advantages of physiological management of the third stage of labour are:
(a) no oxytocic drugs are required;
(b) there is less risk of retained placenta.
The potential disadvantage is an increased risk of post partum haemorrhage.
[B:263; C:192; D:130; I:750]

365 Following signs of separation the usual method

adopted in UK hospitals is the Brandt–Andrews technique. The use and timing of oxytocics prior to the delivery of the placenta is debated but in many hospitals an injection of oxytocin 5 units and ergometrine 0·5 mg is given intramuscularly either with the birth of the anterior shoulder of the child or at the completion of the second stage.
[B:264; C:193; F:124; I:757]

366 One hand of the accoucheur grasps the cord and exerts a constant downward traction, the other hand holds the uterus and pushes the fundus upwards. By controlled cord traction, the placenta usually advances until it is delivered. Care must be taken that the membranes do not tear as they are delivered. The latter may be facilitated by twisting the placenta around a few times, producing a rope effect on the membranes.
[B:265; F:125]

367 Active management of the third stage of labour has the advantages of:
(a) reducing the length of time of the third stage;
(b) reducing blood loss.
It suffers from the disadvantage that unless the placenta is removed from the uterus within 5 minutes, it is likely to be retained. The risk of inadvertently giving an oxytocic before delivery of a second (often undiagnosed) twin is always present.
[A:426; B:263; C:193; D:129; F:124; I:757]

368 Inspection of the placenta is important to check that no portion of it or the membranes are missing and retained in the uterus.
[A:425; B:265; C:195; D:130; I:756]

369 The average weight of the placenta at term is 600 grams—about 1/6 of the weight of the baby.
[A:121; D:52; F:18]

370 In the rhesus-negative mother, cord blood is taken to study the ABO and rhesus group, haemoglobin level, direct Coombs' test and bilirubin level of the baby.
[B:138; D:262; F:450]

371 The umbilical cord should be inspected in order to detect the presence of anomalies. A true knot (very rare) may be a cause of intrauterine growth retardation. The presence of only one artery and vein may be associated with anomalies of the fetus.
[A:573; B:268; C:195; D:270; F:126]

372 Velamentous insertion of the umbilical cord occurs when the vessels of the cord run across a small or large portion of the membranes prior to entering the placenta. In rare cases these vessels may lie in front of the presenting part (vasa praevia) and if ruptured, give rise to bleeding and exsanguination of the fetus.
[A:574; B:266; D:270]

373 A battledore placenta is described when the cord is inserted into the side of the placenta rather than the centre. It is more likely to be torn from the placenta during controlled cord traction.
[A:573; B:40; F:20]

374 A circumvallate placenta is described when the membranes are inserted on the surface of the placenta rather than the edge. It is not of great clinical significance but it is suggested that there is a greater incidence of minor degrees of ante partum haemorrhage with these placentae.
[A:552; B:267; D:30]

375 A succenturiate lobe is a small accessory placenta attached to the main placenta by an artery or vein passing across the membranes. Its significance is that it may be left in the uterus after delivery. The appearance of ragged membranes with vessels leading up to the edge should make one highly suspicious of a retained accessory lobe.
[A:551; B:266; D:30; F:126; I:756]

Obstetric operations—induction of labour

376 There are two main methods of inducing labour:
  (a) medical—intravenous oxytocin, prostaglandins;
  (b) surgical—forewater rupture, hindwater rupture.
Commonly a combination of both medical and

surgical induction is employed using intravenous oxytocin with rupture of the forewaters.
[B:275; C:419; D:388; F:373; I:491]

377 The hindwaters and forewaters are the two compartments inside the amniotic sac separated by the presenting part. In the case of an ill-fitting presenting part, they are in continuity.
[B:275; D:391; I:502]

378 Forewater amniotomy is a procedure which must be performed as an aseptic technique. After cleansing the vulva and vagina, gentle examination of the cervix is undertaken. A finger is passed through the cervical canal and the membranes swept off the lower segment. A hook or sharp instrument is then utilised to grasp and rupture the amnion and chorion. If only a small amount of liquor is released the head may be gently pushed up until 150–200 millilitres escape. Careful note is made of the colour of the liquor. The fetal heart rate must be checked after the procedure.
[B:275; D:391; F:373; I:500]

379 The following problems may be encountered with oxytocic administration: uterine rupture in the multigravid patient; fetal hypoxia due to hypertonia; amniotic fluid embolism; precipitate delivery. It must be remembered that it is not possible to rupture a primigravid uterus with oxytocics even in the presence of cephalopelvic disproportion. Oxytocin also has antidiuretic properties and the infusion of large volumes of electrolyte free fluids (over 4 litres) has caused water intoxication.
[A:789; B:276; C:419; D:390; F:373; I:491]

380 (a) Intravenously. As equally efficient as synthetic oxytocins, their use is limited because of side effects and expense. They may be used intravenously in severe pre-eclampsia and cases of intrauterine death. Nausea, vomiting, diarrhoea and localised cellulitis are common.
(b) Orally. This method is effective in patients with a favourable cervix but has little to recommend it when membrane rupture is equally as effective.

132

(c) Intracervically. Used extra-amniotically in a Tylose gel, it is very effective but the compound is unstable and difficult to prepare and store.

(d) Intravaginally. Used in wax-based pessaries, the method is gaining wide popularity. In those patients with a favourable cervix, labour usually ensues. In those with an unripe cervix, the favourability is usually improved considerably. Problems have been experienced because the rate of release may not be constant.

[B:277; C:420; D:390; I:497]

381 The two major reasons for inducing labour are:

(a) that the extrauterine environment provides a safer place for the baby than the intrauterine environment.

(b) that the life of the mother is seriously endangered if the pregnancy is allowed to continue.

382 The majority of inductions are done for hypertension, prolonged pregnancy, ante partum haemorrhage or intrauterine growth retardation. Other conditions where it also must be considered are: rhesus disease, diabetes, renal disease (worsening), previous unexplained intrauterine death, persistent vomiting, polyhydramnios and patients over the age of 40.

[B:272; C:417; D:388; F:372; I:505]

383 The complications of induction of labour are:

(a) failure of induction—that is failure to deliver the patient who was expected to deliver normally, within 24 hours of the induction time. One should always be able to justify caesarean section in such cases—if one cannot, then there was no indication for induction of labour in the first place.

(b) maternal and fetal infection—especially if labour is prolonged over 24 hours.

(c) unexpected prematurity.

(d) bleeding—from placental site or vasa praevia.

(e) cord prolapse.

(f) uterine rupture from injudicious use of oxytocin.

(g) accidental haemorrhage—with sudden re-

lease of large quantities of liquor causing placental separation as in hydramnios.
(h) amniotic fluid embolism.
[B:277; C:418; D:392; I:481]

384 Induction of labour is contraindicated in cases of major disproportion, malpresentation other than breech, where there has been a previous caesarean section for disproportion or if there is a pelvic tumour. Oxytocics are contraindicated (or used with extreme caution) in cases where there has been a previous caesarean section, grand multiparity and placental insufficiency. Surgical induction is contraindicated in the flexed or footling breech, when the fetus is dead (except in cases of placental abruption) or if the lie is unstable.
[B:275; I:509]

Obstetric operations—episiotomy

385 Episiotomy is a Greek word meaning cutting of the perineal region.
[F:375]

386 The objectives of an episiotomy are:
(a) to prevent damage to the perineum;
(b) to protect the fetus—e.g. premature babies from an unyielding perineum;
(c) to hasten delivery in cases of fetal distress.
[A:430; B:290; D:361; F:375; I:817]

387 It allows controlled delivery of the fetal head, minimises excessive pressure on the fetal head, prevents perineal and vaginal lacerations (which are often difficult to suture) and may help in the prevention of genital prolapse.
[A:430; B:290; F:375; I:818]

388 Episiotomy incision may be median, mediolateral or J-shaped.
[A:431; B:290; D:362; F:376; I:819]

389 The main disadvantages of the mediolateral or J-shaped episiotomy are:
(a) more difficult to repair;
(b) faulty healing is more common;
(c) dyspareunia is not infrequent.
However, extension of these episiotomies is rare

and they are therefore safer to perform than median episiotomies.
[A:471]

390   The median episiotomy is easier to repair and gives a better anatomical result and is seldom painful in the puerperium and rarely gives rise to dyspareunia. Blood loss is also minimal. The disadvantage is that third degree tears are more likely.
[A:431; B:290]

391   (a) Vaginal and perineal skin.
      (b) Bulbocavernosus muscle.
      (c) Superficial and deep transverse perineal muscles.
      (d) Levator ani muscle (only in deep extensive cuts).
      (e) Ischiorectal fossa fat may be exposed in incisions that are deep and lateral.
[B:290]

392   This is a perineal tear that has extended to involve the rectal mucosa.
[A:432; B:358; D:365]

393   Careful suturing under general anaesthesia or regional block is essential. The apex of the tear must be identified. The anal sphincter is usually involved and this must be sutured with interrupted catgut once the retracted ends have been found. Further treatment such as a low residue diet and confining the bowels is outdated and when a bowel action is finally achieved, thoroughly uncomfortable. The patient should be given a faecal softener and encouraged to use her bowels daily.
[A:432; B:359; D:365]

Obstetric operations—instrumental delivery

394   They have blades, a shank, lock and handle. The blades have a cephalic and pelvic curve. The shank is of variable length, the longer being used for midcavity deliveries. Some models are equipped with an axis-traction handle but few practitioners use this now. The shorter shank models are designed as outlet forceps and have a

very rudimentary handle (Wrigley's). Little traction can be applied. Forceps with a fixed lock can only be used to deliver a baby whose head is in the anteroposterior diameter.

A long shanked forceps with a sliding lock is used for rotating the baby's head. Its main feature, apart from this, is the very reduced pelvic curve of the blade (Kjelland's). They are potentially dangerous both to mother and baby, except in very experienced hands.
[A:1041; B:282; D:393; I:626]

395 (a) Delay in the second stage of labour.
(b) Fetal distress in the second stage of labour.
(c) Maternal exhaustion.
(d) Elective.
[A:1044; B:280; C:468; D:395; F:377; I:638]

396 (a) The cervix must be fully dilated.
(b) The bladder must be empty.
(c) Satisfactory analgesia is required.
(d) The position of the occiput must be known.
[A:1045; B:283; C:468; D:396; F:380; I:626]

397 (a) Lacerations to the perineum, vagina, cervix or lower segment of the uterus.
(b) Haemorrhage from lacerations and from an atonic uterus if labour has been prolonged.
(c) Injuries to the baby through poorly applied forceps blades or excessive force.
(d) Failed forceps, usually as a result of unsuspected disproportion, misdiagnosis of the position of the head, incomplete dilatation of the cervix or rarely outlet contraction.
[A:1047; B:288; C:467; D:403; I:653]

398 Abdominal palpation. If any part of the fetal head can be palpated abdominally, consideration should be given to delivery by caesarean section. Although the presenting part may be felt below the ischial spines on vaginal examination, there may be considerable caput formation and the true position of the fetal head may be well above the spines.
[A:1045; C:470; I:626]

399 This is a vacuum extractor—a traction instrument used as an alternative to the obstetric forceps. It adheres to the baby's scalp by suction

and is used in the conscious patient to assist maternal expulsive efforts.
[A:1059; B:288; C:471; D:403; F:391; I:667]

400   In general, the same as for forceps. It cannot be used in face presentations or for the after-coming head of the breech. Full dilatation of the cervix is not so important as with forceps delivery as the cup can fit through a partially dilated cervix, although if delivery is required before full dilatation, caesarean section will usually be preferred. One of its particular uses is in delivery of the second twin if it is a cephalic presentation, and if the presenting part remains high and the cervix begins to clamp down.
[B:289; C:471; D:403; F:392; I:676]

Obstetric operations—caesarean section

401   The major indications for emergency caesarean sections are:
(a) bleeding,
(b) fetal distress,
(c) obstructed labour.
[A:1082; B:298; C:473; D:405; F:396; I:825]

402   The main complications of caesarean sections are:
(a) immediate—haemorrhage; damage to bowel, bladder; anaesthetic problems; Mendelson's syndrome.
(b) delayed—wound infection; chest or urinary infection; deep vein thrombosis and pulmonary embolism.
(c) late—uterine rupture in subsequent pregnancy; adhesions and intestinal obstruction; a complicating factor in later pelvic surgery.
The maternal mortality rate is 10 times higher following caesarean section than for normal delivery.
[B:302; C:473; D:410; F:403; I:853]

403   If a patient has had a previous lower segment caesarean section a good maxim to follow is if the caesarean section was performed for a non-recurring cause such as fetal distress, breech presentation or placenta praevia, a vaginal delivery may be anticipated. If the caesarean section was done previously for a likely recurring

cause such as cephalopelvic disproportion, a repeat caesarean section is likely.
[B:303; C:474; D:410; I:857]

404   Sudden and complete dehiscence of a caesarean section scar may well result in acute generalised abdominal pain and shock and is not difficult to recognise. Often, however, the signs are less dramatic and the following signs are suggestive of scar rupture:
(a) vaginal bleeding especially with a contraction;
(b) arrest of cervical dilatation;
(c) maternal and fetal tachycardia;
(d) disordered uterine action.
(e) ascent of presenting part
Suprapubic pain or discomfort is a notoriously unreliable sign and is of little significance.
[A:863; B:355; C:460; F:323; I:799]

405   The two types of caesarean section are:
(a) lower segment,
(b) classical.
The difference between the two types of operation is the location of the uterine incision. The lower segment incision is a transverse incision in the lower uterine segment and is the incision used in the vast majority of caesarean sections today. The classical incision implies a vertical incision in the upper segment of the uterus. Scar rupture is more likely in subsequent pregnancies if a classical caesarean section has been performed and indeed a previous classical caesarean section necessitates repeat caesarean section in any subsequent pregnancy.
[A:1085; B:295; C:476; F:399; I:826]

406   The main indications for classical caesarean section are:
(a) transverse lie of the fetus especially if membranes have been ruptured;
(b) fibroids or adhesions obscuring the lower segment;
(c) if a post mortem caesarean section is being performed;
(d) if the patient has invasive carcinoma of the cervix.
[A:1093; B:302; C:476; F:402; I:828]

407 Internal podalic version is carried out when a hand is passed through the fully dilated cervix into the uterus to turn the baby from an oblique or transverse lie into the relatively more favourable longitudinal breech presentation. Vaginal delivery may then be achieved.
[B:279; D:413; F:393]

408 Internal podalic version may be performed if external version has failed to establish a longitudinal lie for delivery of a second twin. The patient must always be anaesthetised and it is a potentially difficult and hazardous procedure for both mother and child. Complications include possible uterine rupture, fetal asphyxia and intracranial haemorrhage. Many obstetricians would now favour delivery by caesarean section.
[B:279; D:413; F:393]

E Disorders of labour

Dystocia, augmentation and premature labour

409 Augmentation of labour is a process of intervention aimed at restoring progressive cervical dilatation to a predetermined speed. A number of partograms have been designed incorporating an 'action line'. If the speed of labour is slow, a diagrammatic representation of it as a line on a partogram will approach or cross this action line rather than parallel or diverge from it. In these circumstances, labour can be augmented first by forewater rupture and then by intravenous administration of oxytocics if necessary.
[B:312; C:415; D:124; F:316; I:605]

410 By not allowing labour to exceed 12 hours, maternal and fetal distress are considerably reduced. The incidence of forceps delivery and caesarean section falls dramatically. The most important aspect is early intervention if slowing should occur. Labour is not accelerated but rather returned to normality. There is no place for 'masterly inactivity' in labour.
[A:788; B:311; C:415; D:124; I:571]

411 Prolonged and difficult labour is commonplace in primigravidae and it is this group that often requires active management. However, labour in multigravidae is rarely prolonged but when it occurs it is likely to be due to obstruction. Uterine stimulation in such cases may cause rupture. It is therefore necessary to separate primigravidae from multigravidae when one considers the management of abnormal labour patterns.
[D:350; F:310]

412 In the condition incoordinate hypertonic uterine inertia, the uterus contracts strongly and frequently but lacks fundal dominance. The net result is a failure of progressive cervical dilatation and descent of the presenting part.
[A:792; B:311; C:415; I:569]

413 Hypotonic uterine inertia is commonly described as an abnormal labour pattern where uterine contractions are weak, occur infrequently or cause delay in labour. It is often divided into:
(a) primary hypotonia (inertia) where contractions are abnormal throughout labour and seen more commonly in primigravidae and in the latent phase of labour. It may result from excessive sedation.
(b) secondary hypotonia (inertia) occurring after there has been an interval of normal uterine contractility. It has been suggested that this is a protective action by the uterus against rupture and occurs when there is cephalopelvic disproportion and when labour is prolonged and the patient tired and dehydrated.
(c) incoordinate uterine action. In this condition the contractions are irregular in frequency and strength. In some case the intrauterine resting pressure is raised and the patient complains of persistent pain or discomfort.
(d) incoordinate hypertonic inertia. In other cases there is a reversal of normal uterine action, the upper segment contracting weakly and the lower segment showing persistent hypertonia. Cervical dilation is then distressingly slow.
Many people now believe that inefficient uterine

action in the primiparous patient can be eliminated and that the terms hypotonic and hypertonic inertia representing different clinical entities to be treated in different ways is not valid. Furthermore it is suggested that the term inefficient uterine action be substituted for these terms describing abnormal labour patterns.
[A:792; B:311; C:415; I:569]

414 Primary uterine hypotonia requires that the labour be augmented by forewater amniotomy if membranes are intact, followed by intravenous oxytocics if cervical dilatation does not progress at the rate of 1 cm per hour.

Secondary uterine hypotonia in multiparous patients suggests obstructed labour and careful appraisal of the situation is required. Injudicious use of oxytocics in such patients could cause uterine rupture. If obstruction is diagnosed, delivery should be undertaken by caesarean section. In primiparous patients actively managed from the outset, obstruction or disproportion resulting in secondary uterine hypotonia is rarely seen. The policy of delivery within 12 hours following initiation of an active management policy, by caesarean section if necessary, unless safe vaginal delivery is imminent, will by definition detect the small number of cases in primigravidae where obstruction has occurred.
[D:347; F:314]

415 The condition of incoordinate hypertonic uterine inertia may be overcome by judicious administration of intravenous oxytocics at an early stage. This slows the frequency of the contractions and restores fundal dominance. Only small doses are required and the action has been likened in effect to that of digitalis on a failing heart.

It is, however, difficult to persuade attendant staff that a woman having frequent, prolonged and very painful contractions, requires oxytocics. The criterion for diagnosis is the failure of progress of labour. A patient whose contractions are measured in decibels is often said to be having 'good' contractions. If progress is shown to be halted, they are thoroughly bad contractions and a remedy must be sought immediately.
[C:415; F:317; I:606]

416 Premature labour may be defined as labour ensuing before 37 completed weeks of pregnancy. Premature labour may also be defined in terms of progressive and non-progressive labour. Approximately 40 per cent of cases initially thought to be in premature labour resolve.

417 In approximately 50 per cent of cases there is an underlying contributory factor resulting in preterm labour. In order of frequency the factors are:
(a) ante partum haemorrhage;
(b) fulminating pre-eclampsia;
(c) elective preterm delivery for obstetric reasons, e.g. rhesus disease, diabetes, ante natal fetal distress;
(d) intrauterine death;
(e) congenital abnormalities.
Other factors which may contribute to preterm labour are multiple pregnancy polyhydramnios, uterine abnormality, cervical damage from previous surgery and infection. There is also a higher incidence in lower socioeconomic classes.
[A:931; D:272]

418 Bed rest and sedation is probably the most effective. Several trials indicate that β-sympathomimetic drugs such as ritodrine are of more use than placebo or ethanol but the benefit and risks of such treatment are far from clear. The drugs must not be used if there is intrauterine infection present, if the membranes have been ruptured for any length of time or if there has been an accidental haemorrhage. Treatment is often combined with the administration of corticosteriods to the mother in the hope that the latter will reduce the incidence of respiratory distress syndrome.
[A:932; B:151; C:413; I:957]

Malpresentations and malpositions

419 In a small number of cases, malpresentation is caused by fetal malformations or intrauterine death. In other cases, the increased perinatal mortality rate is a result of prematurity or multiple pregnancy.

142

Malpresentations also predispose to cord prolapse and prolonged and obstructed labour
which are all potent causes of hypoxia.

Manipulative delivery, maternal hypoxia
during general anaesthesia, maternal ketosis
and dehydration will also lead to an increased
perinatal mortality rate.
[C:373]

420 Malpresentations present increased maternal
risks because:
(a) forceps delivery may be required with its
attendant risks.
(b) general anaesthesia may be required for
operative delivery be it forceps or caesarean
section. Prolonged labour may lead to infection, and obstructed labour to uterine
rupture.
[C:373]

421 The commonest malpresentation in labour is the
occipitoposterior position. This occurs in 10 per
cent of all pregnancies at the start of labour.
[A:818; C:374; D:290; I:612]

422 Two factors seem to be mainly responsible for an
occipitoposterior presentation:
(a) the shape of the pelvis,
(b) a deflexed head.
[A:818; B:338; C:374; D:290; F:260; I:612]

423 An occipitoposterior position should be suspected if:
(a) the head is high at full term.
(b) the uterus is slightly concave below the
umbilicus.
(c) limbs are felt both sides of the midline.
(d) the fetal heart is heard out in the flank.
Diagnosis can be confirmed on vaginal examination.
[B:346; C:374; D:290; F:260]

424 Labour in occipitoposterior positions of the fetal
head tends to be more prolonged and painful.
[B:346; C:374; D:290; F:262; I:615]

425 Labour in occipitoposterior presentations may
be more prolonged and painful because the

143

head is deflexed and presents a larger diameter (occipitofrontal) and flexion with rotation takes longer. This also leads to abnormal uterine action and stretching of the lower segment. Because of the paracervical nerve plexus, this stretching leads to pain which is referred into the back resulting in the common complaint in occipitoposterior presentations, of backache. The shape of the pelvis, which is often abnormal, contributes to the long painful labour.
[C:374; F:262]

426 In about 5 per cent of patients with occipitoposterior positions, labour is terminated by caesarean section because of maternal exhaustion or fetal distress. The majority of occipitoposterior presentations however, undergo long rotation to occipitoanterior positions and then progress as normal. 20 per cent will rotate and become stuck in the occipitotransverse position sometimes resulting in deep transverse arrest. 15 per cent undergo short rotation to direct occipitoposterior presentations.
[A:819; B:349; C:375; D:292; F:264]

427 12 per cent of occipitoposterior presentations will deliver spontaneously otherwise treatment depends on the level of the occiput. If this is at the ischial spines or below then rotation anteriorly, by forceps or manually, to the occipitoanterior position may be performed and delivery achieved by lift out forceps. If this presenting part is well below the spines, forceps delivery as an occipitoposterior presentation can be considered. When deep transverse arrest occurs or the presenting part fails to descend, caesarean section is often necessary.
[A:818; B:349; C:375; D:292; F:264]

428 Management of deep transverse arrest of the occiput depends on the level of the presenting part. If at the ischial spines or below and pelvic outlet contraction is ruled out, rotation to occipitoanterior and instrumental delivery may be anticipated. If the presenting part is above the spines and the second stage of labour prolonged, then consideration may well have to be given to at least a trial of forceps in theatre and

probable caesarean section if any problems are encountered.
[A:819; B:347; C:376; F:267]

429 The incidence of multiple pregnancy in Western Europe is 1:80 but this figure may no longer hold true with the widespread use of ovulation inducing drugs such as clomiphene. In West Africa the incidence is about 1:40.
[A:640; B:155; D:316; I:366]

430 Distinguishing a monozygotic (uniovular) pregnancy from a dizygotic (binovular) pregnancy at birth may be difficult. A close examination of the membranes is necessary. This may include microscopy. Monozygotic twins always have their own amnion but share a common chorion. Dizygotic twins have an individual amnion and chorion.
[A:460, B:156, F:178, I:359]

431 Both infants do not present by the head in the majority of twin pregnancies. The incidence is between 40 and 45 per cent but it still remains the most common presentation. Head and breech, breech and head, and breech and breech together account for a further 50 per cent.
[A:659; B:158; D:316]

432 Fetus papyraceus is a condition in which one twin dies early in pregnancy and becomes shrunken and compressed.
[A:652; B:157; F:178]

433 A diagnosis of multiple pregnancy is made clinically when the uterine size is larger than that expected for the gestational age. You should be suspicious in women with a strong family history, in those with hyperemesis gravidarum, those developing pre-eclampsia in the second trimester and those who have been treated with ovulation inducing drugs. A clinical diagnosis can only be confirmed by the palpation of *more than* two fetal poles. The diagnosis is occasionally made embarrassingly (i.e. after the delivery of the first baby!). (Auscultation of two separate fetal hearts is notoriously inaccurate.)
[A:648; B:157; C:397; D:316; F:179; I:368]

434 Other methods available for the diagnosis of twins are:
(a) ultrasonic examination. This is usually very reliable using the β-scan. A second pregnancy may be identified at the time of a threatened abortion and subsequently disappear.
(b) radiology. This is extremely accurate but to be avoided when possible, especially before the third trimester.
[A:648; B:157; C:397; D:316; I:368]

435 Problems that occur more frequently in multiple pregnancy include:
(a) 'anaemia because of increased fetal demands;
(b) hyperemesis gravidarum;
(c) pre-eclampsia (possibly due to the large placental area);
(d) pressure symptoms—varicose veins, oedema, haemorrhoids, striae, abdominal discomfort etc.;
(e) premature onset of labour and/or rupture of membranes;
(f) ante partum haemorrhage—due to both abruption and placenta praevia;
(g) malpresentations and malpositions;
(h) polyhydramnios;
(i) prolapsed cord;
(j) operative delivery;
(k) retained placenta and post partum haemorrhage;
(l) fetal abnormalities.
[A:651; B:159; C:397; D:317; F:181; I:371]

436 Premature labour in multiple pregnancy probably can not be prevented but traditional teaching favours an increased amount of rest from the 28th week onwards. Controlled trials have shown that there is no advantage in admitting all women with multiple pregnancies from the 30th to 36th week as has been advocated. However, many will need admission because of extreme tiredness or the complications of the condition such as raised blood pressure or ante partum haemorrhage.
[A:657; B:159; C:397; D:318]

437 At least one doctor and midwife, a paediatrician

and an anaesthetist should be present at the delivery of twins. Complications with the second twin may occur very rapidly (such as prolapsed limb or cord) and an anaesthetist may be required immediately. For this reason, all patients with multiple pregnancies must have an intravenous infusion during the second stage of delivery.
[A:659; B:351; I:372]

438 The first twin is delivered in the same manner as a singleton whether presenting by the head or breech. The cord must be cut between two clamps to prevent exsanguination of the second twin. A careful vaginal examination is made and the membranes ruptured once the head or breech is presenting at the brim. A longitudinal lie is ensured by an assistant palpating the fetus per abdomen. Uterine contractions are ensured with an oxytocic infusion. This should encourage a normal delivery of the second twin but forceps, vacuum extraction or occasionally breech extraction may be necessary.
[A:658; B:351; F:183; I:372]

439 The dangers to the second twin following delivery of the first include: premature separation of the placenta leading to acute hypoxia; malpresentations and malpositions; prolapse of the cord.
[A:658; B:351; F:183; I:372]

440 If the second twin was found to be lying in a transverse position after delivery of the first, external version to a longitudinal lie should be attempted. If this fails then membrane rupture and internal version to a breech may be considered but if any difficult is encountered, caesarean section should be embarked upon.
[A:658; B:351; F:183; I:372]

441 The incidence of breech presentation is about 2–3 per cent at delivery. However, it is much more common earlier in pregnancy, as many as 25 per cent of babies presenting by the breech at 28 weeks' gestation.
[A:797; B:161; C:381; D:295; F:275: I:386]

442 Aetiology of breech presentation includes:

147

abnormalities of the uterine cavity such as a bicornuate or subseptate uterus or fibroids intruding into the cavity. Primigravidity is also a factor. Fetal causes are more common. Extended legs, multiple pregnancy, polyhydramnios, placenta praevia, prematurity and fetal abnormalities are all associated with the breech presentation.
[A:797; B:161; I:386]

443 A breech presentation may be diagnosed by palpation which should reveal a smooth firm and round mass at the fundus. This is often ballotable. The patient may complain of pain in the right hypochondrium (due to pressure of the hard head against the rib cage) and observe that there are fetal movements in the pelvic area. Auscultation usually reveals a fetal heart heard maximally around the umbilical area. Vaginal examination, ultrasound or radiology will confirm the diagnosis.
[A:798; B:162; C:382; D:296; F:278]

444 The types of breech presentations that may be encountered are:
   (a) extended breech (frank breech)—the legs are extended at the knee joint;
   (b) flexed breech (complete breech)—the legs are flexed as in a head presentation;
   (c) knee or footling breech.
[B:161; D:295; F:276; I:386]

445 Opinions differ widely as to the place of external cephalic version—a manoeuvre usually performed between the 32nd and 34th weeks. The protagonists believe that it reduces the incidence of caesarean sections and the mortality and morbidity associated with breech delivery. The antagonists maintain that the overall incidence of breech presentation at term is not altered and that the procedure has a 1 per cent mortality.
[A:803; B:162; C:384; D:297; F:278; I:389]

446 A vaginal breech delivery should be carried out in a room equipped to perform immediate caesarean section if necessary. An anaesthetist and paediatrician should be present. Failure of descent of the breech at full dilatation is an indication for caesarean section. When the

breech is distending the perineum, an episiotomy is performed and the breech allowed to deliver spontaneously up to the umbilicus. 'Hands off the breech' is a good maxim at this stage! A loop of cord is then pulled down—mainly to avoid traction on the umbilicus and cord compression. The baby is then gently held by the pelvis, thumbs on the sacrum, and when the scapula comes into view, the arms are freed (using Lovsett's manoeuvre). The fetus is allowed to hang by its own weight to encourage flexion and engagement of the head. Following this, the baby is held by the feet and its body swept up over the maternal abdomen and grasped by an assistant who may encourage flexion of the head by suprapubic pressure. Forceps are usually applied to the aftercoming head when the nape of the neck is visible.
[B:328; D:298; F:284; I:392]

447   Ideally only a minute or so delay should occur between delivery of the fetal trunk and head because of the dangers of cord compression by the fetal head in the birth canal. After 1 minute, active steps to aid flexion and delivery must be taken to avoid hypoxia.
[B:330; D:303; F:287; I:392]

448   The Mauriceau–Smellie–Veit manoeuvre is a method devised independently by the three named obstetricians for delivery of the aftercoming head. The left hand of the accoucheur is placed so that the middle finger lies on the baby's suboccipital region and the ring and index fingers on the shoulders. The middle finger of the right hand is placed in the child's mouth and the ring and index fingers over the malar bones. This hand maintains flexion of the head whilst the two combined provide traction. It is certainly a method every obstetrician should learn in case he is faced with a situation where low cavity forceps are not available.
[A:1072; B:331; D:305; I:398]

449   The causes of death associated with breech delivery include hypoxia, due to delay in delivery, cord compression or placental separation and intracranial trauma.
[A:804; C:383; D:306; I:399]

450 The foot and leg may slip through the incompletely dilated cervix and exert pressure on the vagina and rectum. This will induce the desire to push and in a multiparous woman, she may succeed in delivery of the breech as far as the head. Delivery is then obstructed and irreversible brain damage is likely to occur following traumatic delivery of the head through the partially dilated cervix. This complication can be avoided by the judicious use of epidural anaesthesia early in the labour.
[C:383]

451 (a) Face presentation—1 in 500 deliveries;
(b) Brow presentation—1 in 1000 deliveries;
(c) Shoulder presentation—1 in 200 deliveries.
[A:809; D:309; I:404]

452 Face and brow presentations are caused by any factor that favours extension of the fetal head. Extension frequently occurs when the pelvis is contracted or the baby large. Often an abnormal extensor tone is present. Tumours of the fetal neck (thyroid and branchial cysts) and malformations—anencephaly and iniencephaly—are not infrequently implicated (15 per cent). Polyhydramnios by allowing more freedom of movement and extensor tone may also contribute to these abnormal presentations.
[A:809; B:339; D:309]

453 Usually (in 90 per cent of cases) the presenting part (submentobregmatic diameter) undergoes anterior rotation with the mentum rotating under the symphysis pubis. Spontaneous vaginal delivery can be anticipated. In 10 per cent of cases, posterior rotation occurs with the mentum lying in the hollow of the sacrum. Vaginal delivery is not possible and caesarean section is required for delivery.
[A:809; B:342; C:378; I:407]

454 In many cases, spontaneous correction to the vertex occurs in labour but if the malpresentation persists, delivery is best effected by caesarean section, as the brow presents the largest diameter of the fetal skull—the mentovertical (13 cm)—and vaginal delivery is impossible. On occasions, however, if the baby

is small and the pelvis large vaginal delivery may be feasible.
[A:812; C:380; F:273; I:412]

455 The incidence of oblique and transverse lie is about 1:250. It is most uncommon in primigravidae.
[A:813; B:164; C:390]

456 Aetiological factors predisposing towards oblique and transverse lies are: prematurity, uterine malformations, placenta praevia, multiparity, uterine and extrauterine tumours (ovarian cysts and fibromyomata), multiple pregnancy, fetal malformations and polyhydramnios.
[A:813; B:164; D:312; F:290]

457 If a transverse lie is found ante natally, gentle attempts to bring the fetus into a longitudinal lie are made. Placenta praevia must be excluded by placentography (commonly by ultrasound scanning). If the malpresentation persists after the 36th week, the patient may be admitted to hospital until the baby is delivered. Some authorities advocate correction of the lie at 38 weeks with simultaneous amniotomy. Reduction of the fluid volume may help in maintaining the longitudinal lie.
[A:816; B:165; C:391; D:313]

458 Spontaneous rupture of membranes may result in cord prolapse. If delivery is not expedited obstructed labour, fetal impaction and rupture of the uterus is likely.
[A:815; B:336; C:392; F:293]

459 A transverse lie in labour is managed by immediate delivery by caesarean section.
[A:816; B:337; C:392; D:314]

460 Vaginal delivery of a transverse lie may be possible in the case of a second twin when rupture of the membranes and breech extraction may be feasible.
[B:337; D:315]

461 A compound presentation is a condition in which the hand presents in front of or beside the head. It is not as uncommon as some

authorities believe and is compatible with a normal delivery. Tears of the vagina are common.
[A:817; C:392; F:294]

Obstetric emergencies—cord prolapse

462   Cord prolapse may occur when conditions favour an ill-fitting presenting part. Such conditions include prematurity, polyhydramnios, unstable lie, breech presentation, malformations of the fetus, pelvic tumours (fibroids), placenta praevia (minor degrees), pelvic contraction and other fetal malpresentations causing non-engagement of the fetal head. An excessively long cord has been considered contributory. Artificial rupture of the membranes may lead to cord prolapse when the presenting part is not fitting snugly into the pelvis.
[A:836; B:308; C:394; D:320; F:348; I:417]

463   When cord prolapse occurs the presenting part must be pushed up to avoid compression of the cord. The genupectoral position is the traditional one suggested for the patient but is very difficult for the patient to maintain, especially if she needs transporting to an operating theatre. A left lateral position is more sensible with head-down tilt, if available. Rapid filling of the bladder via a catheter may help to stop the presenting part from descending onto the cord.
[B:309; C:395; D:320; F:350]

464   Other measures necessary when cord prolapse occurs include immediate preparations for delivery. If the cervix is not fully dilated, then caesarean section must be undertaken immediately provided the baby is still alive. If the cord is outside the vagina it should be wrapped in moist sterile gauze and replaced in the vagina.
[B:309; C:395; D:320]

465   Following cord prolapse the overall mortality ranges from 20 to 60 per cent depending upon the facilities available and the place where the prolapse occurs.
[B:309; C:395; D:321; F:349]

466 A primary post partum haemorrhage may be
defined as a loss of 500 ml of blood from the
genital tract within the first 24 hours of delivery
of the infant.
[A:877; B:353; C:437; D:354; F:334; I:759]

467 The main causes of primary post partum haemorrhage are retained products of conception,
uterine atony, trauma to the reproductive tract,
coagulation disorders.
[A:878; B:353; D:354; I:760]

468 Uterine atony may occur following prolonged
labour, prolonged use of intravenous oxytocics,
overdistension of the uterus, grand multiparity,
uterine tumours (fibroids), full bladder, failure
to use oxytocics following delivery of the baby.
[A:878; C:438; F:334; I:760]

469 Uterine atony may be overcome by the use of
oxytocics. A single dose of intravenous oxytocin
may be sufficient but more prolonged use of intravenous synthetic oxytocin (Syntocinon) may
be required at a dose of 20–40 units per litre for at
least one hour and, in many instances, much
longer.
[A:880; B:359; D:357; F:336]

470 The patient must be prepared for general or regional anaesthesia. At least 2 units of blood must
be cross-matched and intravenous infusion
commenced. Manual removal of the placenta
must be carried out under aseptic conditions.
With the patient in lithotomy position, the
fingers of the surgeon are inserted into the
vagina and through the cervix. The latter may be
partially closed and dilatation with the fingers
necessary until the whole hand can be inserted
into the cavity. The other hand must control the
uterine fundus externally. The placenta is then
sought and swept off the wall of the uterus and
then removed. If it is considered that membranes or a portion of placenta remains, the
cavity should be examined with large sponge
holding forceps and gentle curettage attempted
with a large blunt curette.
[B:353; C:439; I:766)

471　First and foremost the bladder must be emptied. If this fails to cause the release of the placenta, a hand should be gently inserted into the vagina to see if the placenta or a portion of it is lying there. Gentle traction on the placenta will then usually remove it. If, however, it is found to be retained in the uterus, intravenous fluids, if not already being given, should commence and blood should be taken for cross-matching of at least 2 units. Oxytocics may be necessary if bleeding persists. Preparations must then be made for operative removal under general or regional anaesthesia.

472　Placenta accreta occurs when the trophoblast penetrates through the decidua and attaches directly to the myometrum. There is no natural plain of cleavage and the placenta becomes morbidly adherent. (The latter is often diagnosed by less experienced doctors at the time of manual removal of the placenta, but is seldom the actual case.) It is associated with placenta praevia or previous uterine surgery such as caesarean section, myomectomy (if the cavity is broached) and even strenuous curettage. Profuse haemorrhage is common and emergency hysterectomy may be necessary.
[A:883; B:354; C:440; I:791]

473　The placenta and membranes must be examined to see if they are complete. The bladder must be emptied. If the uterus is soft, manual massaging of it may induce it to contract ('rubbing up a contraction'). If it continues to relax, then intravenous ergometrine should be given. A careful examination of the genital tract must then take place. The vulva and vagina must be inspected for lacerations and bleeding from an episiotomy stopped. Adequate exposure is essential to inspect the upper vagina and cervix. Trauma is much more likely if forceps have been used, particularly of the rotational type. If bleeding has been excluded from the vulva, vagina and cervix, then a uterine cause must be sought.
[B:359; C:438; I:765]

Uterine rupture; impacted shoulders; uterine inversion, defects of coagulation

474　(a)　Previous surgery particularly caesarean section. Classical scars are much more likely to rupture than lower segment. It is not common after myomectomy but uterine perforation during curettage may lead to a weak spot on the uterus.

(b) Uterine overdistension such as multiple pregnancy and polyhydramnios.

(c) Obstructed labour. This is usually seen in multigravid patients on the rare occasions in which it occurs. Injudicious use of intravenous oxytocics may precipitate the rupture.

(d) Operative trauma. This again is rare but rotational forceps represent the greatest hazard.

[A:862; B:354; C:459; D:367; F:322; I:796]

475 Laparotomy must be performed. In the case of lower segment rupture, this is usually slight and primary repair can be undertaken. In all other cases, hysterectomy is usually necessary to save the life of the patient.

[A:872; B:356; C:460; D:369; F:325]

476 Shoulder dystocia occurs when there is obstruction to the passage of the shoulders through the bony pelvis usually as a result of delivery of an unusually large baby. Severe birth asphyxia or fetal death may occur if delivery is not prompt.

The most important principle of management is to create as much space as possible posteriorly. The patient is immediately placed in lithotomy position and a large episiotomy performed—bilaterally if necessary. The position of the fetal back should be ascertained and fundal pressure applied by an assistant. At the same time the anterior shoulder should be digitally rotated under the symphysis (adducting the shoulder to minimise the presenting diameter). Should this fail the patient should be anaesthetised and the posterior fetal arm grasped, flexed and brought through the pelvis posteriorly. The baby is then rotated through 180 degrees and the other arm delivered in a similar manner.

[A:813; B:323; D:327]

477 Uterine inversion occurs when the fundus of the uterus descends through the cervix and lies in the vagina or outside the

introitus. The placenta is usually still adherent. It is often caused by injudicious cord traction with an atonic uterus.
[A:888; B:360; D:359; F:326]

478   When presented with a case of uterine inversion an immediate attempt to reduce the inversion manually should be carried out. The patient is often shocked and appropriate measures should be taken. Once this has been carried out and if the initial attempt to reduce the inversion has failed, the patient should be anaesthetised and 2 litres of warm saline should be rapidly infused into the vagina. Reflux of fluid is prevented by an assistant using the labia to encircle the accoucheur's right hand which holds the inverted uterus in the vagina.
[A:888; B:360; D:360; F:326]

479   Severe placental abruption is the most common cause. Intrauterine death, especially if the fetus has been dead for more than 4 weeks, may cause the condition. Amniotic fluid embolism is a rare and often fatal cause. Severe sepsis and severe eclampsia may occasionally lead to the condition.
[A:493; B:199; C:306]

480   An amniotic fluid embolism is the entry of amniotic fluid into the maternal circulation via maternal venous sinuses. The fluid will contain fetal hair, vernix, squamous cells, and, when lodged in the pulmonary circulation, may cause severe respiratory embarrassment. They act as thromboplastins.
[A:519; B:366; C:465]

481   There is a massive release of extrinsic thromboplastins into the circulation leading to rapid depletion of fibrinogen. This, in itself, may lead to failure of clotting. Occasionally, fibrin degradation products (FDPs), which are lytic in themselves, may worsen the condition. Treatment with transfused fibrinogen will then be like adding fuel to the fire. The best remedy is fresh blood transfused as soon as possible. Heparin, as an intravenous loading dose of 10 000 units, will prevent further intravascular coagulation and fibrinogen levels will be restored.
[A:519; B:366; C:306]

F The puerperium

482 The puerperium is the period following completion of the third stage of labour until return to the normal non-pregnant physiological state 6 weeks later.
[A:457; B:370; D:131; I:862]

483 Involution is the return of the reproductive tract to its normal non-pregnant state. There are catabolic changes leading to breakdown of muscle tissue and gradual diminution in the size of the uterus over a period of 6–8 weeks.
[A:457; B:370; C:197; F:127]

484 The lochia is the passage of blood clot, decidua, leucocytes and trophoblastic tissue from the placental site which is shed from the genital tract during the first 4–8 weeks. It is initially red (lochia rubra) for the first 10 days or so then becomes a yellow serous discharge (lochia serosa) for 3–4 weeks. Finally it becomes white (lochia alba).
[A:465; B:370; C:197; D:132]

485 Colostrum is the first milk produced by the milk glands before birth and for several days after. It is yellow in colour but rich in proteins, cells, minerals and vitamins. Most importantly it contains large amounts of immunoglobulin antibodies which give the baby resistance to infection in the early months.
[A:462; B:371; D:138; F:473]

486 In most mammals, prolactin is essential for milk synthesis and secretion. It appears to exert two actions on mammary tissue—mammatrophic and lactogenic. Prolactin levels are greatly elevated at full term and failure of lactation is a result of inhibition by high levels of oestrogen and progesterone. After delivery loss of these placental steroids remove this inhibition and milk secretion occurs.
[A:462; B:407; C:198; D:138; F:473]

487 Most spontaneous abortions occur in the first trimester and lactation does not occur. This is probably a result of inadequate hormone preparation of the breasts. Lactation may,

however, follow second trimester abortions and suppressive therapy may be necessary.
[F:473]

488 Following delivery basal levels of prolactin fall but in breastfeeding patients they remain throughout lactation at levels above those found in non-pregnant women. In addition, there is a prompt surge in prolactin secretion in response to nipple stimulation during suckling. This lasts approximately 30 seconds in the early puerperium and concentrations are related to the quantity of milk produced. During established lactation less prolactin is released at suckling but its effects are amplified by an increase in prolactin receptors in the areolar cells.
[A:464; C:198]

489 Many students are aware of the summing-up often used for the advantages of breastfeeding, namely: it's at the right temperature; it contains exactly what the baby needs; it's bacteria free; it comes in cute containers and the cat can't get at it! There is, however, no doubt that the proportion of water to other constituents in breast milk is exactly right to prevent dehydration and constipation. The protein content of breast milk is 1·2 per cent—less than cows' milk but more easily digestable. It also contains the specialised proteins—immunoglobulins which carry antibodies from the mother and afford protection to the baby in the early months. The antibodies in cows' milk are effective against cows' diseases but not human ones! The fat, carbohydrate and mineral composition is also ideally suited to babies' needs.
[B:407; I:898]

490 The high lactose, low phosphorous and protein levels in breast milk prevent the growth of certain organisms such as *E. coli* and dysentery. The breast-fed baby's gut also contains *Lactobacillus bifidus* which is encouraged to grow by a special nitrogen-containing sugar—the bifidus factor found only in breast milk. These organisms produce acetic and lactic acid which also prevent the growth of many disease-producing organisms.

Breast milk also contains lactogenin which together with IgA immunoglobulin inhibits the growth of *E. coli*, yeasts and staphylococci by robbing them of room for growth. Three other factors interact to kill bacteria—lysozyme, immunoglobulin A and complement. Breast milk also contains an anti-staphylococcal factor, hydrogen peroxide and vitamin C which together kill bacteria. It also contains an enzyme lactoperoxidase which inhibits bacterial growths. Other substances which are not antibodies but act against certain viruses such as polio, mumps and encephalitis have also been found in breast milk.

491 There are very few contraindications to breastfeeding, the main one being if the mother does not wish to breastfeed, or the baby is for adoption. If the mother has open tuberculosis, poorly controlled epilepsy or a puerpural psychosis, breastfeeding is again contraindicated. Breast abscesses requiring surgery would also be a contraindication as well as any drugs transmitted in breast milk which may be harmful to the baby—for example tetracyclines, antithyroids, cytotoxics and steroids.
[B:413; F:479]

492 Lactation can be suppressed by impairing the secretion of prolactin or inhibiting its action on the breast. Therefore, avoiding nipple stimulation reduces prolactin secretion. This together with supporting the breasts and simple analgesia are the traditional methods of natural suppression of lactation. The most certain way of reducing milk formation is by pharmacologically inhibiting prolactin secretion using bromocriptine. The administration of oestrogen orally or by injection is effective but considerably increases the risk of venous thrombosis.
[A:918; B:415; C:453; D:144]

493 The definition of puerperal infection is a temperature of 38 °C on any two days occurring within 14 days of abortion or delivery.
[A:894; B:384; D:372; I:877]

494 The incidence of infection in the puerperium is

approximately 3 per cent, but any patient with a pyrexia must be investigated. The genital tract is usually the site of infection in 25–55 per cent of cases, the urinary tract in 30–60 per cent, the breast in 5–10 per cent of cases and at other sites in 2–5 per cent.
[A:895; B:384; D:372; I:878]

495 All investigations of puerperal pyrexia begin with a thorough history. A look at the ante natal record will determine if the infection was present before labour, whether she had a urinary tract infection, was anaemic or had a vaginal infection. The obstetric record will reveal how long the membranes were ruptured and whether the liquor was offensive and the type of delivery and extent of genital tract lacerations.

A general physical examination will include the throat, lungs, heart, breasts, abdomen, legs (to exclude venous thrombosis) and perineum with particular note taken of the character and nature of the lochia.

Special investigations should include a speculum examination and high vaginal swab, a gentle bimanual examination to detect abnormal pelvic tenderness or swellings and a midstream specimen of urine for microscopy and culture and haemoglobin and white cell count. If septicaemia is suspected a blood culture should also be taken.
[A:902; B:384; D:372; I:887]

496 The organisms responsible may be introduced from exogenous sources or may be normal inhabitants of the genital tract. In the majority of cases the organisms arise from the bowel and commonly inhabit the lower genital tract. In 70 per cent of cases anaerobes as well as aerobic organisms are found. The commonest anaerobes are *Bacteroides, Streptococcus* and *Clostridium*. The commonest aerobes are *E. coli, Staphylococcus* and haemolytic *Streptococcus*.
[A:899; D:373; F:415; I:878]

497 In non-breastfeeding mothers menstruation returns on average 8–10 weeks after birth. In breastfeeders the average length of time varies according to whether breastfeeding is partial or complete. In a mother who totally breastfeeds

for 6–8 months and continues with the breast for drinks and comfort when the baby starts solids, the average length of time for resumption of menstruation is 14 months. It also varies with the nutritional state of the mother—the less well nourished mothers have a later onset of menstruation following delivery.
[A:469; C:197; D:133]

498 A woman is less likely to conceive while breastfeeding. Lactation, however, is accompanied by only a moderate contraceptive effect, it is temporary and of low reliability. 40–75 per cent of breastfeeding women resume menstrual function while still nursing.
[A:469]

499 It would appear that the elevated prolactin levels in the breastfeeding mother inhibit the response of the ovaries to follicle stimulating hormone. Ovulation therefore is impaired.
[A:469]

500 Cracked nipples may be treated by the use of soothing oils or ointments. Deeper cracks will mean resting the nipple and gentle expression of the milk to maintain the supply.
[B:373; F:422]

501 Urinary complications that may arise in the puerperium are:
(a) urinary retention—commonly occurs following delivery due to bruising of the bladder base and/or discomfort from the episiotomy or vaginal tear. The bladder easily becomes overdistended, holding a litre or more of urine and resulting in retention with overflow.
(b) suppression of urine—a volume of less than 500 ml in the first 24 hours is usually a result of the more serious complications of pregnancy—septic abortion, placental abruption, severe pre-eclampsia, disorders of coagulation, amniotic fluid embolism, water and electrolyte depletion or abnormal responses to drugs.
(c) urinary incontinence—stress incontinence not infrequently follows delivery but is seldom marked in the early puerperium. Continuous leakage may be a result of

fistula formation following instrumental delivery and occurs immediately following delivery. If the fistula results from prolonged pressure of the fetal head on the bladder in labour sloughing and incontinence occur 8–12 days later.

(d) urinary infections—one of the chief causes of puerperal pyrexia. It may be a recurrence of earlier infection in pregnancy or acquired as a result of urinary retention and catheterisation.

[A:468; B:386; C:448; I:820]

502　The likelihood of venous thrombosis in late pregnancy and the puerperium are increased due to three factors—infection, stasis of blood and alterations in its constituents. Infection usually occurs at delivery and spreads to the pelvic side wall. Venous return is retarded from the calf in late pregnancy and the puerperium. This is even more evident in patients who have had prolonged bed rest as a result of pregnancy complications both before and after delivery. There is also a considerable rise in platelet and fibrinogen concentration.

A further factor of importance is the administration of oestrogens to suppress lactation. There is a reported tenfold increase in venous thrombosis in women over 25 years of age if this method is used. It is probably not a direct cause but an additional factor sufficient to tip the scales in patients who by reason of age, parity, operative delivery or past history are more likely to develop this complication.

[A:908; B:200; C:443; I:906]

503　Prophylactic measures that may be undertaken during pregnancy to prevent thrombosis occurring are:

(a) during pregnancy—the prevention of anaemia and treatment of varicose veins.

(b) during labour—the avoidance of exhaustion, dehydration and haemorrhage; the avoidance of trauma to limbs from the pressure by stirrup rods when in lithotomy position and pressure under the knees while in Trendelenburg position. Also bruising of the limbs in moving the unconscious patient should be avoided.

(c) during the puerperium—early ambulation;

the avoidance of sitting in Fowler's position (with legs hanging over the chair or
bed impeding venous return); and by
regularly inspecting the legs to detect the
earliest signs of thrombosis in susceptible
patients.
[B:201; C:446; D:380]

504 Approximately 3 per cent of patients in the
puerperium will develop venous thrombosis.
Superficial venous thrombosis is commonest
occurring in 2 per cent of patients. Deep vein
thrombosis occurs in 1–2 per cent of patients.
[B:386; D:378]

505 In superficial thrombosis the treatment is
usually rest and application of ichthyol and
glycerine dressings. Resolution usually occurs
in 2–4 days.
   The management of deep venous thrombosis
is essentially anticoagulant therapy—Intravenous heparin followed by either subcutaneous heparin or oral anticoagulants (warfarin)
for 6 weeks. Elastic support and rest of the
affected limb is practised until pain has
resolved. Following this ambulation is
encouraged.
[A:908; B:386; C:446; I:908]

506 The object of the post natal examination is to
detect and rectify any abnormal condition resulting from the recent pregnancy, labour or
puerperium. By treating minor ailments, much
suffering and chronic ill health will be prevented.
[B:373; D:148; F:131]

507 The most likely cause is retained fragments of
placental tissue which may or may not be
infected. Curettage will usually be diagnostic
and curative but chorionic gonadotrophin
assays should be considered if there is any
doubt over the diagnosis, as on rare occasions,
choriocarcinoma may present in such a
fashion.
[C:450; D:358]

G Maternal and perinatal mortality statistics

508 A maternal death is one that can be attributed

to pregnancy or childbirth. Definitions vary from one country to another. In the United Kingdom, deaths up to one year after birth or an abortion are considered. The definition used by the Federation of International Gynaecology and Obstetrics excludes deaths more than 6 weeks after delivery or abortion.
[C:491; F:518]

509 The most common causes of maternal death in England and Wales between 1973 and 1975 were:
(a) hypertensive disease,
(b) pulmonary embolism,
(c) abortion,
(d) haemorrhage,
(e) caesarean section.
The largest number of deaths occurred with caesarean section but some of these were due to anaesthetic complications or from haemorrhage, pulmonary embolus or sepsis. For the first time abortion was no longer the single most common cause of death in the Report on Confidential Enquiries into Maternal Deaths between 1973 and 1975.
[B:86; D:425; F:519]

510 The main reasons for the improvement in maternal mortality rates are:
(a) the discovery of antibiotics;
(b) the availability of blood transfusion and flying squad services;
(c) improved maternity hospital services;
(d) improved medical standards;
(e) improved social conditions.
[C:491; F:518]

511 The perinatal mortality rate is defined as the number of stillbirths (born after 28 weeks) together with the number of neonatal deaths in the first week of life per 1000 total births. However, if an infant is born before 28 weeks' gestation and shows signs of life but then dies, it is classified as a neonatal death.
  The International Classification of Diseases (ICD) ninth version, suggests that PMR should include infants weighing more than 500 g or those with a gestational age of at least 22 completed weeks or a crown–heel length of at least 25 cm.

512 Latest figures available indicate the PMR in England and Wales to be 13·5 per 1000 births.

513 The main causes of perinatal death are:
(a) prematurity,
(b) congenital anomalies,
(c) hypoxia,
(d) birth trauma,
(e) haemolytic disease,
(f) infection.
[B:93; C:501; F:525]

514 The factors influencing perinatal mortality are:
(a) birth weight—the lower the birth weight the higher is the perinatal mortality. This applies to premature and small for gestational age infants.
(b) social class—the lower the social class the higher the perinatal mortality.
(c) maternal age and parity—the perinatal mortality is lowest in women between the 20 and 30 years age group. Following this time it increases steadily and is three times the norm at the age of 40. Mortality rates also increase with the fourth and subsequent pregnancies.
(d) race—the mortality rate in the UK is increased in women from India, Bangladesh and the West Indies (but not among those from Pakistan).
(e) multiple pregnancy—the perinatal mortality rate is increased for multiple births.
(f) smoking—although difficult to quantify, there is little doubt that smoking leads to low birth weight infants and increased risk of ante natal and intrapartum hypoxia.
[C:502; D:428]

H The neonate

515 The average baby's birth weight in Europeans is 3·2 kg. and the average head circumference at birth is 35 cm.
[B:400]

516 It is a system of scoring the condition of a newborn infant at 1 and 5 minutes. Five parameters are used, namely colour, respiratory

165

effort, heart beat, muscle tone and reflex ir-
ritability. Each is given a score of 0, 1 or 2. A
lively baby with no evidence of depression will
get a score between 7 and 10—a severely depressed infant in need of intensive resuscitation between 0 and 3.
[B:424; D:453; F:463]

517   If a baby is born in poor condition or fails to
      breathe within 1 minute of birth, active resus-
      citation may be required. If, at 3 minutes,
      respiration is still not established and the heart
      rate less than 60 beats/min assisted ventilation
      is required. An Apgar score of 6 or less at 5
      minutes suggests a degree of birth asphyxia.
      Babies who fail to show any signs of spon-
      taneous respiration after 20 minutes of active
      resuscitation have a very poor prognosis.
      [B:423; D:453; F:463]

518   Meconium aspiration can result in a fatal
      pneumonitis. Babies born at risk of meconium
      aspiration must be prevented from gasping
      and inhalation of liquor at birth by a firm
      two-handed grasp of the baby's chest wall
      immediately on delivery. Any meconium
      present must be aspirated from the naso-
      pharynx and larynx under direct vision.
      [A:959]

519   Gestational age of the infant can be judged
      independently of menstrual history by assess-
      ing neurological and physical criteria of the
      newborn infant. This is known as the
      Dubowitz score. A further scoring system
      based on physical characteristics, namely skin
      texture, lanugo hair, ear form and firmness,
      genitalia, breast size, nipple formation and
      plantar skin creases, known as the Parkin score
      may also be useful. These scoring systems
      however, only provide an approximation
      which may differ from the true gestational age
      by at least 2 weeks in either direction.
      [B:435]

520   Babies of birth weight 2500 g or less are
      classified as low birth weight. There are two
      categories of low birth weight babies.
      (a) preterm—which defines those babies born
          before 37 completed weeks but who are

of average weight for their gestational age.
(b) small-for-dates—which defines those babies
having a birth weight below the 10th centile
for the gestational age.
[B:435]

521 The clinical features noted in premature babies
are:
(a) the skin is red, thin and covered with
lanugo hair;
(b) the head appears large compared to the rest
of the body;
(c) the ear cartilage is poorly developed;
(d) the breast tissue is poorly developed;
(e) the plantar skin creases are poorly
developed;
(f) the labia minora are prominent in females
and testes undescended in males.
Babies who have suffered from intrauterine
growth retardation often have the wizened old
man appearance and are dehydrated. There is
little if any subcutaneous fat and the skin is dry,
cracked and peeling and may also be stained
with meconium.
[B:437; D:468]

522 The problems of premature babies which may be
encountered may be classified as:
(a) respiratory problems—respiratory distress
syndrome; apnoeic attacks.
(b) hypothermia.
(c) inability to suck and swallow.
(d) jaundice.
(e) infection.
(f) intraventricular haemorrhage.
The problems of small-for-dates infants are as
follows:
(a) respiratory problems—severe birth asphyxia; pulmonary haemorrhage;
pneumonia.
(b) hypoglycaemia.
(c) hypothermia.
(d) polycythaemia.
(e) intrauterine viral infection.
(f) congenital abnormalities.
[B:443; D:469]

523 Babies may be labelled as having respiratory distress if they have at least two of the following
signs after the age of 4 hours:

167

(a) respiratory rate greater than 60,

(b) costal recession,

(c) grunting.

It must be remembered that a baby presenting with tachypnoea may have an abnormality unrelated to lung disease such as cardiac abnormalities or methaemoglobinaemia. Other main causes of respiratory distress are as follows: hyalin membrane disease, meconium aspiration, pneumonia, pulmonary haemorrhage or hypoplasia and pneumothorax.
[B:431; F:466]

524 The general principles involved in the treatment of an infant with HMD are as follows:

(a) nurse in an incubator and maintain adequate temperature control;

(b) minimal handling is necessary;

(c) regular observations of oxygen concentration, respiratory and heart rates;

(d) oxygen therapy if required—initially continuous positive airways pressure (CPAP) or intermittent positive pressure ventilation (IPPV) if necessary.

CPAP is usually instituted in those babies whose clinical condition is poor and whose respirations are grossly irregular and in those babies requiring more than 60 per cent oxygen to achieve arterial oxygen tensions of greater than 60 mmHg.
[A:958; B:433]

525 Excess oxygen is poisonous. Concentrations above that found in air (20 per cent) are unsafe if breathed for long periods. If arterial oxygen content remains too high for too long retinal capillaries will be damaged and retrolental fibroplasia occurs. The preterm baby is particularly at risk. Bronchopulmonary dysplasia may also follow prolonged oxygen therapy resulting in chronic pulmonary insufficiency. Both these conditions may be prevented by careful monitoring of arterial oxygen and incubator oxygen tensions and limiting oxygen therapy to those situations where it is really necessary.
[A:960; B:445]

526 Jaundice is commonly seen in the neonate for the following reason. *In utero* the baby's unconjugated bilirubin is removed by the placenta.

After birth, conjugation must occur in the baby's liver and in every baby there is a rise of serum bilirubin in the first days of life after which time the level should fall.
[B:472]

527 Causes of jaundice that have to be considered in the neonate are:
(a) haemolytic disease;
(b) ABO incompatibility;
(c) infection and dehydration;
(d) large haematoma or extensive bruising;
(e) breast milk jaundice (it is suggested some mothers excrete a steroid in their breast milk which aggravates jaundice by competing with bilirubin for conjugation),
(f) some drugs (e.g. sulphonamide, vitamin K analogues, salicylates, diazepam);
(g) other rare causes such as cretinism, galactosaemia, hepatitis and bile duct atresia.
[B:473]

528 Jaundice in the newborn requires investigation or action when:
(a) jaundice is visible in the first 24 hours of life—this suggests haemolysis;
(b) jaundice that is severe at any stage;
(c) jaundice that seems to be improving but recurs or jaundice that appears after the fourth day; this suggests infection, dehydration, or one of a number of rare diseases;
(d) jaundice which persists for more than 7 days (unless rapidly fading).
[B:473]

529 The methods available for reducing serum bilirubin levels are:
(a) exchange transfusion;
(b) phototherapy blue light (this converts the bilirubin in skin to biliverdin which is water soluble and harmless);
(c) phenobarbitone—induces the activity of glucuronyl transferase required for the conjugation of bilirubin. Its use and value are debatable at present;
(d) Adequate fluid and food intake.
[B:477]

530 Kernicterus occurs in babies whose serum unconjugated bilirubin reaches high levels. In

such circumstances unconjugated bilirubin crosses the blood–brain barrier inhibiting essential enzymes and causing brain damage. With ideal neonatal management, kernicterus should rarely if ever occur.
[A:974; B:472]

531 These antibodies cannot cross the placenta and therefore must have been produced by the baby. They are therefore evidence that the baby has been infected *in utero*.
[B:467]

532 Ortolani's test is performed in order to detect congenital dislocation of the hip. The Guthrie test is used as a screening test of phenyl-ketonuria (PKU). In PKU there is a deficiency of phenylalanine hydroxylase which converts phenylalanine to tyrosine. This leads to mental retardation and high levels of phenylalanine in the blood which may be detected in blood samples obtained from heel prick—Guthrie test.
[D:450]

GYNAECOLOGY

A Anatomy of the female reproductive organs

533 The vulva consists of:
  (a) mons pubis
  (b) clitoris
  (c) urethral orifice
  (d) vestibule
  (e) labia majora
  (f) labia minora
  (g) vaginal orifice
  (h) hymen
  (i) bulb of the vestibule
  (j) Bartholin's glands.
[E:19; G:1; H:1; J:17]

534 The vestibule is the area between the labia minora and is perforated by the urethral and vaginal orifices and the ducts of Bartholin's glands.
[G:2; H:2; J:18]

535 The perineal body is the fibromuscular area

between anus and vagina giving rise to the attachment of 8 muscles: sphincter ani, bulbospongiosus, 2 superficial transverse perinei, 2 deep transverse perinei and 2 levator ani muscles.
[G:25; J:20]

536 The relations of the uterus are as follows:
(a) anteriorly—the upper part of the uterus has the uterovesical pouch and either intestines or bladder in front. The lower part is directly related to the base of the bladder.
(b) posteriorly—the pouch of Douglas, posterior fornix and coils of intestines.
(c) laterally—the broad ligament and uterine artery running up the side of the uterus giving off branches. As it passes forward to reach the base of the bladder, the ureter lies only 1 cm to the side of the cervix and passes under the uterine artery to reach the bladder.
[E:27; G:4; H:6; J:25]

537 The main supports of the uterus are the fibromuscular condensations of tissue in pelvic fascia:
(a) uterosacral ligaments,
(b) transverse cervical ligaments (Mackenrodt's cardinal ligaments).
[E:27; G:28; H:8; J:43]

538 The ovaries receive their blood supply directly from the abdominal aorta via the ovarian arteries.
[E:32; G:16; J:44]

539 The right ovarian vein normally joins the inferior vena cava, but the left ovarian vein usually drains into the left renal vein.
[E:32; J:47]

540 The first step in normal sexual differentiation is the establishment of genetic sex. Secondly, under the control of genetic sex the gonads differentiate, determining the hormonal environment of the embryo, the differentiation of the internal duct systems and the formation of the external genitalia.
[C:1; E:34; H:164; J:155]

541 The primitive gonads are bipotential, the medulla being a potential testis and the cortex a potential ovary. Differentiation into a testis depends on the active influence of the Y chromosome. This produces an antigen which causes medullary development and cortical regression. This antigen is known as the Y induced histocompatibility antigen. In the absence of a Y chromosome, the gonad becomes an ovary about two weeks later than testicular development.
[E:34; H:164]

542 The Wolffian and Müllerian ducts are discrete primordia which temporarily coexist in all embryos. One type of duct persists giving rise to special ducts and glands whereas the other disappears during the third fetal month.
[E:34; G:29; H:170; J:128]

543 Androgens from the early testicle stimulate development of the Wolffian duct into epididymis, vas deferens and seminal vesicles. Another substance—as yet unidentified—the Müllerian inhibiting factor (MIF) is responsible for regression of the Müllerian duct system in the male. In the absence of a Y chromosome and lack of MIF, the Müllerian system develops into the fallopian tube, uterus and upper vagina, while in the absence of testosterone, the Wolffian system regresses.
[E:34; H:170; J:130]

544 In the bipotential stage the external genitalia consist of a urogenital sinus, two lateral labioscrotal swellings and a genital tubercle. In the presence of a Y chromosome and androgen production, the genital tubercle forms the penis, the labioscrotal folds fuse to form a scrotum and the folds of the urogenital sinus form the urethra. In the absence of a Y chromosome (i.e. in the presence of an ovary or absence of gonad) the urogenital sinus remains open forming the labia minora, the labioscrotal folds form the labia majora and the genital tubercle forms the clitoris. The urogenital sinus develops into the vagina and urethra. Thus the lower vagina is formed as part of the external genitalia.
[C:4; E:35; H:173; J:133]

B Physiology of menstruation

545 The hypothalamus, pituitary and ovaries.
[E:50; G:34; H:17]

546 Increasing levels of follicle stimulating hormone (FSH) are released from the anterior pituitary under the influence of gonadotrophic releasing hormone (GnRH) from the hypothalamus. The increasing amounts of FSH promote follicular development in the ovary and, in turn, increasing oestrogen production.
[E:50; G:34; H:20; J:64]

547 After the FSH fall prior to midcycle there is still a further rise in oestrogen levels. By positive feedback there is a sudden release of GnRH which leads to a massive surge of luteinising hormone (LH), from the pituitary (there is a smaller rise in FSH at the same time). This surge of LH causes follicular rupture and ovum release about 24–30 hours later.
[E:57; G:35; H:24; J:69]

548 Oestrogen and progesterone. They arise from the luteinised theca-granulosa cells. If conception fails to occur the levels fall and menstruation results. There is a compensatory rise in FSH and a new cycle begins.
[E:60; G:39; H:28; J:71]

549 There is a negative feedback to the hypothalamic pituitary axis. Increasing levels of oestrogen cause a fall in GnRH and hence FSH levels.
[E:57; G:37]

550 It causes an active development of the myometrium and changes the prepubertal organ into its adult size. The endometrium undergoes proliferation, stimulating the growth of the glandular component. The cervix becomes softer as oestrogen levels increase and the cervical columnar glands increase their production of mucus.
[E:52; G:46; H:38; J:59]

551 The vagina becomes more vascular and the epithelial and muscular elements grow. The epithelial cells become filled with glycogen.

Glycogen, in turn, is broken down by lactobacilli (Döderlein's bacilli) which cause a lowering of vaginal pH. This acidity protects the vagina and uterus from invasion by pathogenic organisms.
[E:53; G:46; H:38; J:60]

552 It has no effect unless the endometrium has been initially primed by oestrogen. When this is the case, the proliferative endometrium undergoes secretory changes. The stroma becomes oedematous, the glands fill with glycogen-rich mucus and proliferation is arrested.
[E:54; G:47; H:46; J:62]

553 17-β-Oestradiol (E2), oestrone (E1), and oestriol (E3). Oestradiol is transported to tissues bound to albumin where it is taken up by target cells. These are mainly found in organs derived from the paramesonephric duct and also in the breast. Further metabolism of oestrogens occurs in the liver where they are conjugated with glycuronic acid and excreted mainly in the urine.
[E:52; G:45; H:37]

554 Spiral arteries arise at right angles to the basal arteries that course through the myometrium. In their course through the basal layer they are straight but become progressively coiled as they rise through the endometrium. As the endometrium thickens they are able to lengthen. Just prior to menstruation, progesterone levels fall and there is shrinkage of the endometrium due to fluid loss. This leads to coiling of the arteries with resultant diminished blood flow leading to hypoxic and necrotic changes of the superficial and intermediate layers. Shortly after, the straight portions of the arteries go into spasm for long durations with resultant necrosis of the overlying tissues. Short phases of vasodilatation cause surges of blood through the arteries which separates the necrotic layers and removes them from the uterine cavity. The blood which initially clots undergoes lysis and is expelled along with the endometrium. Only the basal layer remains. Average loss is between 50 ml and 80 ml per cycle.
[E:63; G:38; H:56; J:76]

555 During the follicular or proliferative phase, exfoliated cells are mainly superficial squamous cells. They are large and flat with pyknotic nuclei. As the cycle progresses and under the influence of progesterone, more intermediate cells are apparent. The edges of the squamous cells tend to turn in giving an envelope effect and later in the cycle the cells roll up—the navicular stage. Pus cells are plentiful and the squamous cells tend to clump together.
[E:68; H:70]

C   Disorders associated with the menstrual cycle

556 It is a variety of symptoms suffered by a minority of women, usually in their fourth decade. These symptoms tend to commence about 7 days prior to the onset of menstruation and are relieved by menstruation. In some patients symptoms may develop almost immediately after ovulation. The syndrome is characterised by some or all of the following symptoms: mastalgia, a feeling of bloating, heaviness of the lower abdomen, headaches, changes in bowel function and most disturbingly, emotional changes. The latter may be a display of unusual aggression, irrational behaviour, depression and lethargy. Criminal acts are said to occur far more commonly in the premenstrual phase.
[E:71; G:262; H:825; J:547]

557 It has been considered that changes in oestrogen, and progesterone balance are the most important factors. However, serial measurements of these hormones have failed to reveal any standard pattern in sufferers. Hypersecretion of aldosterone may also play a part.
[E:71; H:825]

558 The use of progestogens or pure progesterone is often the most successful approach. Dydrogesterone given in the latter half of the cycle is effective for many women especially when given in conjunction with a mild diuretic. Much success has been claimed for pure progesterone vaginal pessaries (200–400 mg a day) premenstrually. Some patients, especially those who suffer from

175

headaches and depression react favourably to pyridoxine in doses ranging from 40 mg to 100 mg a day. A compassionate doctor willing to listen to the patient and prepared to help is often a major help on the path to recovery.
[E:72; H:826; J:548]

559 This condition is similar to PMS but weight gain is usually more dramatic and oedema easily demonstrated. Salt free diets are helpful and the diuretic spironolactone 50 mg–100 mg a day for 7 days premenstrually is often effective.
[E:73; H:827]

560 Painful menstruation. Three types are recognised, namely spasmodic (or primary); congestive (or secondary); and membranous, the latter characterised by acute colicky pain and the passage of an endometrial cast. Membranous dysmenorrhoea is most uncommon.
[E:72; G:259; H:817; J:537]

561 The pain occurs with the onset of menstruation and usually lasts for the first day only. It is colicky in nature and the pain may radiate from the lower abdomen to the inner aspects of the thighs. There is often associated nausea and vomiting. The condition is usually seen in girls in their late teens and early twenties, who are nulliparous. It is far more common amongst girls living in institutions (and this includes nurses' homes). Maternal attitudes may be an important factor.
[E:280; G:260; H:817; J:538]

562 Numerous treatments have been advocated. The aetiology of the condition is unknown but uterine ischaemia has been implicated. Similarities between primary dysmenorrhoea and migraine have been sought and treatment with drugs such as clonidine advocated. High circulating levels of prostaglandins may be one of the causes and drugs such as flufenamic acid are useful if started early enough. Analgesics such as aspirin or codeine may provide symptomatic relief. There appears to be a strong relationship with ovulatory cycles in many sufferers and treatment with the combined oral

contraceptive pill may produce remission of symptoms. Where the pill is unacceptable, treatment with synthetic progestogens for 3 weeks may give good results. Surgery is not advocated. Enthusiastic dilatation of the cervix may provide temporary relief of up to 6 cycles but is not curative and may leave the cervix permanently damaged. Presacral neurectomy was once advocated but is never performed nowadays.
[E:280; G:261; H:821; J:539]

563 This condition is characterised by a prolonged dull constant pain in the lower abdomen and back. It usually starts 3–4 days before menstruation and may continue until the cessation of bleeding. The common causes are endometriosis, pelvic inflammatory disease and pelvic congestion. Treatment is that of the primary cause.
[E:73; G:259]

564 Literally, middle pain. This is pain induced by ovulation, and is therefore constant in its timing in relationship to the cycle. The pain is thought to arise through peritoneal irritation by blood escaping from the ruptured follicle. Paradoxically, it often occurs only on one side and may be sufficiently acute to warrant hospital admission. Many normal appendices have been removed by eager (and inexperienced) young surgeons who have mistaken the diagnosis and failed to take an accurate menstrual history.
[E:68; H:828; J:544]

565 This is a term used to categorise abnormal menstrual patterns, when organic diseases have been excluded. It includes various or unknown causes of heavy menstrual loss (menorrhagia), frequent periods (epimenorrhoea) and prolonged bleeding (metrorrhagia), or a combination of two or more.
[C:565; E:74; G:252; H:777; J:517]

566 Most simply, into anovulatory and ovulatory bleeding. In the first case there may be insufficient follicular development or impaired positive feedback to the hypothalamus (and pituitary). Polycystic ovary syndrome is

177

another cause. In ovulatory abnormal bleeding, an inadequate luteal phase may be the cause but in many cases the basis of the abnormal pattern is unknown.
[C:566; H:784, 788; J:523]

567   A careful history is most important, bearing in mind the age of the patient, the presence of other symptoms, her desire to start or further her family and the severity of her symptoms. The latter is perhaps the most difficult as it may be hard to quantify menstrual loss and it is up to the patient to describe what she considers abnormal. However, her haemoglobin level is a good indicator of excessive loss. Examination should include a note of her weight (in relation to her height), her blood pressure, any evidence of endocrine disease and signs of a bleeding tendency. Pelvic examination may reveal an enlarged or tender uterus, evidence of endometriosis or fixed retroversion. Endometrial curettage is mandatory in a woman over 35 years of age, either as an inpatient or outpatient. Other investigations such as a hysterogram, laparoscopy, hysteroscopy or laparotomy are, on rare occasions, necessary. A full blood picture and possibly coagulation screen are of considerable use.
[C:582; E:77; H:778; J:527]

568   In the first instance, endometrial curettage. This must be considered diagnostic but on occasions (up to 30 per cent) it is curative. After correction of anaemia, further therapy can be divided into hormonal, non-hormonal and surgical.
[C:584; E:78; G:256; H:790; J:530]

569   The most commonly used is progestagenic therapy. This may take the form of norethisterone, dydrogesterone or medroxyprogesterone acetate used cyclically in courses of 5–21 days for up to one year. In cases of cystic endometrial hyperplasia, this is often curative. In younger women, particularly those under the age of 30, combined oestrogen–progestogen preparations as found in the contraceptive pill may be indicated. Those with abnormal bleeding patterns who are subfertile may be helped by ovulation inducing agents

such as clomiphene citrate and tamoxifen. In those with polycystic ovary syndrome, additional therapy with prednisone can be helpful.
[C:585; E:80; J:531]

570 This is a condition characterised by a variable period of amenorrhoea, usually 6–8 weeks, followed by heavy, continuous and painless menstrual bleeding. It is found at either end of reproductive life but is more common nearer the menopause. It is a feature of anovular cycles in which oestrogen levels are high. Diagnosis can only be made by curettage.
[C:573; E:80; J:526]

571 The endometrium is hyperplastic and in the proliferative phase. The glands are of variable size and some are very considerably larger than usual, giving rise to the characteristic 'Swiss cheese' appearance.
[E:80; H:382]

572 Curettage may be curative itself and, in the short term, is the case with metropathia haemorrhagica. However, the procedure must be considered primarily as diagnostic. If hormonal therapy fails, then hysterectomy must be considered. However, this should only be undertaken when a patient has completed her family and should not be undertaken lightly. In recent years, it has almost become a fashionable operation and many surgeons may find themselves pressurised by the patient herself. Many unjustified stories surround hysterectomy, especially postoperative depression, obesity and loss of libido. These can be avoided provided there is proper patient selection, the procedure is explained and any myths which are unfounded dispelled by careful counselling.
[C:589; E:81; J:532]

573 This condition, which by definition can only occur six months after the cessation of menses, is relatively common and may be caused by oestrogen therapy, atrophic changes of the vagina and cervix, endometrial or cervical malignancy, cervical polyps, endometrial hyperplasia and, rarely, hormone-producing

ovarian tumours, and bleeding from the urinary or alimentary tract mistaken for vaginal bleeding. In about one-quarter of cases no cause is found.
[E:288]

574 Apart from a history and careful clinical examination diagnostic curettage is mandatory, even when an obvious cause may be apparent (e.g. an endocervical polyp). This must be done to exclude intrauterine neoplasia.
[E:289]

575 The patient is placed in the lithotomy position and the vulva, perineal and perianal area cleaned with a suitable antiseptic (e.g. povidone-iodine solution). The vagina and cervix are cleaned in a similar manner. The patient is draped with sterile towels. The cervix is visualised by placing a speculum in the vagina and is grasped with a tenaculum. A sound is passed through the cervical os to gauge both the length and axis of the uterine cavity. With the use of progressively larger dilators, the cervix is dilated and narrow polyp forceps introduced. They are opened and closed whilst rotating them through 90° and any polyps removed. A sharp curette is then inserted to the fundus and withdrawn with firm pressure on the uterine wall. This is repeated in a radial fashion until the entire cavity is curetted and the endometrium thus obtained is sent for histological examination. The whole procedure is usually carried out with general anaesthesia.

576 Cervical malignancy must always be considered of prime importance. Endocervical polyps and, rarely, cervical erosions can cause occasional bleeding. Vaginal infections, particularly *Monilia*, may give rise to the condition. Other causes will include breakthrough bleeding when the patient is taking oral contraception and various causes of an unstable endometrium. Except in rare instances (breakthrough bleeding in the young), curettage should be undertaken. Cervical cytology is essential.

D Intersex

577 (a) Phenotype—this is the external appearance

of the person and is usually dependent upon the external genital organs.

(b) Psychological or gender sex—this is the gender that the person asigns to himself or herself. It is dependent usually upon the phenotype and the sex in which that person has been brought up.

(c) Gonadal sex—this is dependent upon the gonad that is present. There are conditions in which the phenotype may be female and the gonad testes and vice versa.

(d) Chromosomal sex—the absence of a Y sex chromosome will always create a female genotype, even in circumstances when there is only a single X chromosome, as in Turner's syndrome (45XO).

[C:37; E:46; H:209]

578 This is known as congenital androgen insensitivity (previously called testicular feminisation). The end organs of the body are totally insensitive to androgens and the result is a phenotypical female. There usually is no axillary or pubic hair and the vagina is very short. The uterus and tubes do not develop because of Müllerian inhibition. The patient has testes, usually found in a hernial sac in the inguinal canal or occasionally in an intra-abdominal position. They need to be removed surgically because of the risk of malignant change. The patient who is sterile, is always assigned the female sex and should never be told the diagnosis.

[C:43; E:49; G:73; J:171]

579 In this condition, the primordial germ cells fail either to develop or to migrate to the gonad. The gonads are streaks of tissue containing no follicles. The patients are of a female phenotype and have a rudimentary uterus and tubes. Breast development may be poor but can be enhanced by cyclical administration of oestrogens. (The contraceptive pill is a convenient way of giving this.) In Turner's syndrome (45XO) the patient has a short stature, webbed neck, cubitus valgus and may be mentally subnormal.

[C:41; E:48; G:71]

580 This condition occurs when a female fetus

(chromosomally and gonadally) is subjected to androgens *in utero*. It may occur as a result of congenital adrenal hyperplasia or the mother ingesting androgens during pregnancy. In either case, the external genital organs will become masculinised, to a greater or lesser extent.
[C:45; G:73; H:216; J:166]

581 There may be labial fusion to form a scrotum. Clitoral hypertrophy may occur. Later the urethra may become incorporated into the clitoris to give varying degrees of epispadias or hypospadias.
[C:45; H:216]

582 This is a syndrome in which a male has one or more extra sex chromosomes, the most common being XXY. They are usually tall, infertile males with small testes and occasionally gynaecomastia. The syndrome is caused by paternal chromosomal non-dysjunction.
[C:40; H:227; J:163]

E   Amenorrhoea, virilism and hirsutism

583 Amenorrhoea is the absence of menstruation. It may be primary, being a failure to menstruate by the age of 16, or secondary, occurring when a woman who has previously menstruated fails to do so for more than 3 months.
[E:82; G:244; H:733; J:498]

584 Pregnancy and ovarian failure (the menopause).

585 This is an unusual cause of primary amenorrhoea. Regular menstruation exists but escape of the menstrual blood is prevented by an occluding membrane of the vagina at the level of the hymen. (The hymen itself can be seen lying on the membrane and the condition is not caused, as was thought, by an imperforate hymen.) The membrane is at the level of the junction between the urogenital sinus and Müllerian ducts.
[C:10; G:78; H:200; J:143]

586   The patient is usually around the age of 14 or 15. There has been normal development of breasts and secondary sexual hair growth. The patient may present with primary amenorrhoea, an abdominal mass and retention of urine. A history of monthly lower abdominal pain may be obtained. On examination the patient has a distended bladder. Vaginal examination will reveal the bulging membrane which may have a bluish coloration. Retention of urine is due to the accumulated blood grossly enlarging and elongating the vagina, which, in turn, stretches the urethra to such an extent that micturation becomes impossible. Treatment is by urethral catheterisation followed by incision of the membrane under general anaesthesia.
[E:40]

587   Polycystic ovary syndrome, ovarian failure, absent or inappropriate gonads (Turner's syndrome and androgen insensitivity syndrome).
[C:53]

588   These may be classified as hypothalamic, pituitary, gonadal and other diseases including thyroid and adrenal disease. The most frequent conditions accounting for almost half the cases (when pregnancy and the menopause have been excluded), are hyperprolactinaemia and weight loss.
[E:84; G:245; H:734]

589   Age and previous menstrual history are of obvious importance. Recent emotional upsets should be asked about. A history of weight loss, medication, hot flushes and galactorrhoea are very relevant and general questions relating to other endocrine disorders may be helpful. Occasionally patients may complain of increased hirsutism.
[C:56; H:735]

590   The two most important tests are an assessment of follicle stimulating hormone (FSH) levels and prolactin (PRL) levels. If FSH levels are very high, this suggests ovarian failure (or absence). Moderately raised levels and high luteinising hormone (LH) levels suggest polycystic ovary syndrome. Low FSH (and LH) levels indicate a hypothalamic or pituitary disorder. If prolactin

levels are very raised (four times the laboratory upper level) a pituitary tumour must be excluded. This can be done by radiography of the pituitary fossa, computerised tomography (CAT scan), visual field assessment and, occasionally, carotid arteriography or air encephalography.
[C:57; G:249; H:735]

591   The progestogen withdrawal test. After administration of a suitable progestogen for about 3–5 days, a withdrawal bleed will occur 3–7 days later if the endometrium has been exposed to adequate levels of oestrogen. However, failure of bleeding could indicate a uterine abnormality as well as low oestrogen levels.
[H:736]

592   In a patient who does not wish to become pregnant, no treatment is necessary. If she wishes to have regular periods there is no contraindication to her starting a low dose oral contraceptive preparation. In those wishing to attain a pregnancy there are three lines of treatment. Those who have low FSH and LH levels and a progestogen withdrawal bleed, will usually respond to clomiphene citrate given for 5 days in doses from 50 mg to 200 mg a day. Those with raised LH levels (polycystic ovary syndrome) may respond to small doses of clomiphene citrate with added prednisone at a dose of 2·5 mg three times a day throughout the cycle. Those patients with low FSH and LH levels who fail to respond to the progestogen withdrawal test usually fail to respond to clomiphene citrate (but this should be tried) They will need therapy with human menopausal gonadotrophins to induce ovulation.
[C:63; E:88; H:739]

593   Inappropriate galactorrhoea. This is present in about a third of cases of women with raised prolactin levels. The patient may not be aware of it but gentle squeezing of the breast may demonstrate it.
[C:57; E:84; H:747]

594   A pituitary tumour (usually a microadenoma), raised thyrotrophin levels, drug therapy (especially phenothiazines, tricyclic antidepressants, oral contraception), hypothalamic

lesions (meningitis and encephalitis). Remember that breast stimulation and stress can raise prolactin levels. Blood should therefore be withdrawn when the patient is at rest and not immediately after a physical examination.
[C:59]

595 Provided that pituitary tumour has been excluded (see above) and other causes are not apparent, the patient may be commenced on bromocriptine, a dopamine agonist. Initial side effects such as vertigo and nausea can be minimised by starting on a low dose (1·25 mg a day) and increasing it every 3 days until a response is obtained. A dose of 2·5 mg twice or three times a day is usually sufficient.
[C:62; G:251; H:750]

596 The patients may have some or all of the following problems: obesity, hirsutism, anovular cycles or amenorrhoea, virilism, polycystic ovaries.
[C:60; E:83; H:744]

597 Mild cases of adrenogenital hyperplasia, ovarian and adrenal tumours, Cushing's disease and polycystic ovary syndrome.
[C:71]

598 The most useful investigation is measurement of the free plasma testosterone level. 17-Oxosteroid concentration in urine is most unreliable as large amounts of any adrenal androgen must be present for it to be raised. If available, androstenedione and dehydroepiandrostenedione levels are of use. Patients with amenorrhoea should be investigated as outlined earlier. In cases of adrenal hyperplasia, androgen levels will be depressed dramatically if dexamethasone is administered. This will not occur if a tumour is present.
[C:75]

599 In many cases, no cause is found and it must be considered as a variation of normality. When adrenal or ovarian tumours are present, then surgery is necessary. Steroid suppression is usually effective in cases of adrenal hyperplasia. Where the cause is considered to be

dysfunctional and fertility is not a problem, then reversed sequential therapy with cyproterone acetate and oestrogen given cyclically is effective if continued for a year or more. Where this drug is not available, small doses of steroids or the contraceptive pill may be helpful. If fertility is required and anovular cycles are present (polycystic ovary syndrome), treatment with clomiphene citrate and prednisolone usually restores ovulation. Very occasionally wedge resection of the ovary is necessary.
[C:76]

F Abortion, ectopic pregnancy and trophoblastic disease

600 The term refers to expulsion of the conceptus, either spontaneously or therapeutically, before it reaches a state of viability. In the UK this is at the conclusion of the 28th week of gestation but it is likely that this definition will change soon. The World Health Organization recommends that the fetus be considered viable when its gestational age is in excess of 20 weeks or when it weighs more than 400 grams. This has been adopted in parts of the USA and Australia.
[C:203; E:135; G:289; J:187]

601 The commonly quoted figure is 15 per cent of all pregnancies. However, it seems highly likely that many other pregnancies abort at or about the time of the expected menses and therefore go unnoticed.
[C:203; E:135; H:727; J:187]

602 The majority are as a result of malformation of the conceptus or defects in its implantation. Maternal causes include systemic disease, particularly viral infections; uterine abnormalities such as bicornuate uterus or fibromyomata that distort the cavity; and cervical incompetence, giving rise to midtrimester abortion. Stress and emotional problems are said to play a part in some cases.
[C:203; E:135; H:719; J:189]

603 Spontaneous abortions can be subdivided into

threatened, inevitable, incomplete, complete, missed and septic. Therapeutic abortion means a termination of the pregnancy surgically or by medical induction within the laws of the country concerned. The term abortion has unfortunately come to mean therapeutic termination of pregnancy in the eyes of most non-medical people, who refer to spontaneous abortion as a miscarriage.
[C:210; E:137; G:293]

604   In this condition, the patient complains of a red or brown vaginal loss. There is seldom acute pain but a period-like discomfort is common. On clinical examination, the uterine size is compatible with the gestational age and the cervical os is closed. Continuing viability of the pregnancy should be confirmed by urine pregnancy test and, where available, ultrasonic examination of the uterus. Treatment is, by tradition, confinement to bed but it is doubtful that it plays any major part in conserving a pregnancy. Drug treatment is best avoided. There is no evidence that progestogens, by whatever route, make any difference to the outcome. In early pregnancy (between 5 and 8 weeks) repeated injections of HCG may help to conserve or boost progesterone production by the corpus luteum.
[C:210; E:138; G:293; H:727; J:193]

605   With either, the patient will complain of fresh bleeding and pain. The pain is colicky in nature and lower abdominal. On pelvic examination in an inevitable abortion, the cervical os will be dilated and the conceptual sac may be felt bulging through. The uterine size is compatible with the gestational age of the pregnancy. The findings are similar with an incomplete abortion but the patient is usually aware that she has passed something or products of conception may be found in the vagina. The uterine size may be smaller than the age of the pregnancy or occasionally larger, if distended by a blood clot.
[C:211; E:139; G:294; H:728; J:194]

606   The patient should be moved to hospital and the necessary precautions taken in case of major haemorrhage. There is seldom any place

for conservative management. The patient must be examined vaginally and if products are found in the vagina or cervical os, they should be removed with sponge-holding forceps. If bleeding is heavy, intravenous or intramuscular ergometrine 0·25 mg to 0·5 mg can be given. The patient must be examined under general anaesthesia and the uterine cavity gently curetted with a large curette. This is a potentially dangerous procedure and should not be delegated to the most junior member of the team except when under supervision.
[C:212; E:139; J:195]

607 Haemorrhage and infection. The former can occur if prompt action is not taken with an incomplete abortion or heavy loss is not anticipated. The latter is a complication less frequently seen in the UK since the introduction of legal abortion, as it frequently was the consequence of illegal abortion carried out by unskilled people in unsterile circumstances. Septic abortion may occur if there is excessive delay in evacuating a uterus following incomplete abortion.
[C:212; H:728]

608 The patient is pyrexial and has a tachycardia. There is often a purulent offensive vaginal discharge. The uterus is boggy and tender and the cervical os open. There may, in severe cases, be evidence of pelvic or generalised peritonitis or even endotoxic shock. The most common organisms involved in septic abortion are usually endogenous such as *Streptococcus faecalis, E. coli, Bacteroides, Proteus*. Occasionally *Clostridium welchii* may be present.
[C:219; E:140; G:296; J:198]

609 A high vaginal swab and blood culture should be taken prior to therapy in an attempt to identify the organism responsible. Treatment is started with suitable antibiotics such as gentamicin and metronidazole. Provided severe haemorrhage does not supervene, curettage may be delayed for 12 hours or more from the commencement of therapy.
[C:219; E:141; J:200]

610 This is a situation in which the pregnancy fails

to survive but is not expelled spontaneously. The patient may complain that she no longer feels pregnant and clinical examination will reveal a uterus whose clinical size is smaller than that expected. Subsequent examinations at weekly intervals will confirm a uterus failing to enlarge or even decreasing in size. Immunological tests of pregnancy will remain positive whilst there is surviving trophoblast but these will in time become negative. Ultrasonic examination will confirm the diagnosis. There is no urgency for treatment but if the conceptus is not spontaneously aborted after a reasonable length of time, treatment should be instituted. When the uterus is less than 14 weeks' size, cervical dilatation and suction curettage should be carried out. When the uterus is larger, oxytocics must be used. Extra-amniotic prostaglandin is a suitable and safe treatment.
[C:212; G:298; H:727]

611   It is said to be between 20 and 25 per cent. If a patient has three or more successive abortions she is said to be a habitual aborter.
[C:217; E:144; H:718]

612   In approximately one-third of patients, there appears to be no antecedent factor. In the remainder there is usually a history of cervical injury caused by previous delivery through a partially dilated cervix; dilatation and curettage; vaginal termination of pregnancy; cone biopsy; Manchester repair.

613   (a) Any patient who has had a previous midtrimester spontaneous abortion for unknown reasons, must be suspected. The history usually reveals spontaneous expulsion of the conceptus with relatively little pain.
    (b) Dilatation of the cervical os greater than 2 cm in the midtrimester of pregnancy strongly suggests cervical incompetence.
    (c) Any patient in the non-pregnant state whose cervical os will accept a Hegar No. 8 dilator with minimal resistance probably has the condition.
    (d) All patients who have undergone previous wide dilatation of the cervix (in excess of Hegar No. 12) for termination of pregnancy

189

or who have had a large cone biopsy must be suspected as having a potentially incompetent cervix. Subsequent repeated cervical examination in pregnancy will reveal the condition, if present.
[C:213; E:144; G:299]

614   By the introduction of a cervical encircling suture early in the mid trimester. This was first introduced by Shirodkar and in many centres the suture still bears his name, although the technique for its introduction bears little resemblance to his original description.
[C:214; E:144; J:203]

615   She must remain in bed for 3–4 days after its introduction. After mobilisation, she may go home but must rest. She may have increased bladder frequency and a vaginal discharge. She must be told that if she experiences pain, bleeding or rupture of the membranes, she must report to hospital immediately. Under normal circumstances the suture will be removed in the 38th week of pregnancy.

616   The safest method is by dilatation of the cervix and suction curettage using a hollow curette of appropriate diameter (usually no more than 10 mm) made of soft plastic, glass or metal. The earlier the termination is performed, the safer the operation is.
[C:206; E:145; G:300]

617   This procedure is most safely carried out by the use of prostaglandins (E_2 or $F_{2\alpha}$) either extra- or intra-amniotically. When used intra-amniotically they may be combined with hypertonic solutions such as urea or used in higher concentrations alone. Formally intra-amniotic hypertonic saline or hysterotomy were performed but are rarely used now.
[C:209; G:304]

618   It is a pregnancy that implants outside the uterine cavity. The most common site is the fallopian tube but it can occur in the cervix, in the cornu of the uterus, on the ovary or in the abdominal cavity. Over half ectopic gestations occur in the ampulla of the tube and not more than 2 per cent at any site other than the tube.
[C:222; E:235; G:306; H:636; J:207]

619 This is largely unknown but factors delaying the passage of the fertilised egg down the tube must be responsible in most cases. It seems likely that previous infection is a major cause and there is an increased incidence amongst IUCD users and those patients taking progestogen-only pills for contraception.
[C:223; G:306; H:636; J:208]

620 (a) Tubal abortion may occur, resulting in either its total absorption or its extrusion into the peritoneal cavity or its incomplete extrusion with subsequent intraperitoneal blood loss or occasionally, the formation of a tubal mole (a large haematoma contained in the tube).
(b) Tubal rupture may take place in one-third of cases and this is associated with rapid blood loss and its sequelae.
(c) Rarely, secondary abdominal implantation can occur.
[C:224; E:236; G:308; H:639; J:210]

621 Any woman in the reproductive phase of life who gives a history of lower abdominal pain and amenorrhoea should be suspected of having an ectopic pregnancy. However, amenorrhoea may not occur in one-fifth of cases and an immunological test of pregnancy may well be negative. If bleeding occurs, it is usually brownish and watery (described by some as looking like prune juice) and follows the onset of pain. It marks the sloughing of the endometrium (decidua). The subsequent pattern may be acute or subacute.

In acute cases, the patient may have evidence of acute peritoneal irritation with marked pain, abdominal rigidity and rebound tenderness. She may complain of fainting and display evidence of impending shock (tachycardia and hypotension). If intraperitoneal blood loss is extensive it may track along the paracolic gutter to the underside of the diaphragm. This gives rise to the classical sign of right shoulder pain. Vaginal examination gives rise to acute pain and movement of the cervix can only exacerbate the discomfiture and should not be done. Every precaution to treat massive blood loss must be taken if an ectopic pregnancy is suspected.

In subacute cases, the pain may be dull, or acute but of short duration. There is usually tenderness of the lower abdomen and vaginal examination reveals a fullness in one or other fornix. Movement of the cervix from side to side may produce pain.
[C:224; E:238; H:644; J:212]

622 (a) Acute appendicitis, especially when the appendix is pelvic. In these circumstances there may be unusual uterine bleeding.
(b) Rupture of a corpus luteum cyst.
(c) Uterine abortion.
(d) Pelvic infection.
(e) Torsion of an ovarian cyst or fallopian tube (hydrosalpinx).
[E:240; J:213]

623 As stressed already, the necessary precautions against massive concealed haemorrhage must be paramount in the mind of any doctor dealing with a case of suspected ectopic pregnancy. If the patient's general condition is good and clinical signs are sufficiently vague to preclude the making of a definite diagnosis, the patient should be examined under general anaesthesia. In the absence of any pelvic findings, laparoscopy is the surest way of confirming the diagnosis. If a tubal pregnancy is present, then immediate laparotomy should be undertaken. Salpingectomy (either total or partial, depending upon the site of pregnancy) is carried out. Much debate has surrounded the advisability of removing the ipsilateral ovary but most authorities feel that it is unnecessary.
[C:226; E:239; H:651; J:215]

624 Immediate resuscitation must be carried out by replacing lost intravenous fluid but there must be the minimal of delay in getting the patient to an operating theatre and stopping the bleeding. Further resuscitation with cross-matched compatible blood can then be undertaken.
[C:227; G:314]

625 About one in ten. There is also a high incidence of subsequent infertility, with about 40 per cent of patients failing to conceive again.
[E:241]

626 Trophoblastic disease. There is a large spectrum

of changes ranging from simple hydropic degeneration, through hydatidiform mole to frank malignancy with choriocarcinoma.
[C:229; E:210; G:202; H:659; J:220]

627　In European countries and the USA, the incidence is 1 : 2000 pregnancies but in South Asia it occurs with considerably greater frequency (1 : 300 to 1 : 600). It is most frequently found in primigravidae and also multigravid women over the age of 40, usually of low socioeconomic grouping.
[C:234; E:210; H:660; J:221]

628　Much interest has surrounded the karyotype of hydatidiform moles, which are almost always 46XX. Of considerable note has been the discovery that the entire chromosome content of the mole comes from the sperm.
　　There is duplication of the haploid (23) chromosomes of an X-bearing sperm which then fertilises an ovum, causing ejection of the ovum nucleus along with the second polar body whose formation is delayed until the time of sperm entry. This is also called androgenesis.
[C:231; H:665]

629　The first sign is usually vaginal bleeding similar to that of a threatened abortion. However, it tends to occur early in the second trimester (around 14th–18th week of pregnancy). Occasionally, grape-like vesicles may be expelled. The uterine size is commonly greater than that expected for the gestational age. Hyperemesis is a frequent feature and pre-eclampsia occurs in a quarter of cases, the larger the uterine enlargement the greater the incidence. The uterus has a soft doughy consistency and the fetal heart is absent. Serum or urinary gonadotrophin levels are markedly raised. Luteal cysts are a consequence of this rise in chorionic levels. An interesting feature is the development of thyrotoxicosis in some cases.
　　Diagnosis can be confirmed by the use of ultrasound; there is a typical 'snow-storm' appearance.
[C:234; E:221; G:204; H:670; J:223]

630　There are three main lines of treatment,

namely oxytocic stimulation, suction curettage and total abdominal hysterectomy. Oxytocic stimulation has, for many years, been the most popular method but is now giving way to suction curettage. The immediate danger of any form of evacuation is haemorrhage and the necessary precautions must be taken. Many authorities advocate repeat curettage about 5 days after the initial evacuation to remove any remaining trophoblastic tissue. Hysterectomy has been considered advisable for women over the age of 40 or who have completed their family. With the advent of successful chemotherapy, this is no longer thought to be so necessary.
[C:236; E:222; H:679; J:224]

631 Serum or urinary levels of HCG can now be measured by radioimmunoassay (and differentiated from LH by the β-subunit). These should be done initially on a weekly, then monthly basis and finally 3-monthly basis as levels begin to fall. An initial chest X-ray is also useful.

The patients must be seen and evidence of malignant change sought (such as abnormal bleeding or respiratory complications). Chemo-therapy must be carried out if there is evidence of metastases, a sudden rise or a failure to fall in the HCG levels. If the levels fall to normal then, if the patient wishes, a further pregnancy may be undertaken after one year has elapsed. Safe contraception is mandatory whilst HCG levels are falling and the oral contraceptive pill seems ideal but reports suggest that this might slow down the fall in HCG levels and increase the incidence of malignant change. The intrauterine device, therefore, seems the most ideal, despite the problems of intermenstrual bleeding.
[C:237; H:680]

632 It occurs after hydatidiform moles in 40–50 per cent of cases, after abortion in 25–40 per cent of cases and after normal pregnancy in 10–25 per cent of cases. It can, very rarely, coexist with a normal pregnancy. Its incidence is between 1:10 000 to 1:30 000 depending upon the area of the world in which it occurs. The time interval between the pregnancy and its appearance varies from immediate to many years.
[E:222; H:668; J:228]

633 The most common sign is irregular vaginal bleeding after a pregnancy. Sometimes this may be massive. Metastases may present as lumps in the vulva or vagina, or give rise to respiratory symptoms such as haemoptysis. Direct invasion through the myometrium may lead to intra-peritoneal haemorrhage. Amenorrhoea may be a feature when metastases produce HCG in quantities sufficient to supress the hypo-thalamopituitary–ovarian axis.
[C:238; H:672; J:229]

634 Prior to the introduction of chemotherapy, the survivial rate following surgery with or without radiotherapy was practically nil. However, chemotherapy now offers survival rates between 80 and 100 per cent depending upon the volume of tumour present and the time interval between the onset of the disease and the initi-ation of treatment. The folic acid antagonist methotrexate is widely used either alone or in combination with drugs such as actinomycin D and 6-mercaptopurine. Near lethal doses have to be given and therefore should only be under-taken in highly specialised centres. Surgery is indicated as an adjuvant to chemotherapy where haemorrhage is uncontrollable.
[C:239; E:223; G:205; H:681; J:230]

635 This is a tumour lying midway between hydatidiform mole and choriocarcinoma. The condition is usually locally invasive and distant metastases are rare. The distinctive feature of the invasive mole is the excessive trophoblastic proliferation into the myometrium. Treatment is by chemotherapy and, once again, surgery is only indicated if there is massive intraperitoneal haemorrhage.
[H:667]

G Diseases of the vulva

636 Itchiness of the vulva. It is one of the more commonly seen (and mis-spelt) problems in gynaecology. It is suggested that about a third of cases may have a psychosomatic origin but before that diagnosis can be made, it is essential that other causes are excluded.
[C:654; E:158; G:114; H:247; J:558]

637   (a) Generalised disease such as diabetes or jaundice. Oestrogen deficiency may be an important factor in the postmenopausal patient.

     (b) General skin diseases like psoriasis, fungal infections, scabies etc. may cause pruritus vulvae. Very occasionally, threadworms may migrate from the anus to the vulval area.

     (c) Allergies. It is suggested that some patients may become allergic to various detergents or nylon underwear. Any tight clothing, such as trousers and jeans, will cause an increase in sweating in the area and exacerbate the problem. All patients with pruritus should be encouraged to wash their underwear in soap, use cotton rather than nylon pants, replace their tights with stockings and wear skirts or dresses rather than trousers or jeans.

     (d) Vaginal discharges such as monilial infections and to a lesser extent trichomonal infections are the most common cause of pruritus. Clinical examination, microscopy of the discharge and bacteriology will confirm the diagnosis and the appropriate action can be taken.

     (e) Psychosomatic disorders. Already mentioned, these may be the cause in a minority of patients. Mental disorders or psychosexual problems may underlie the condition.

638   If the pruritus is long standing, a vulval biopsy is necessary to exclude dysplasia. Advice about clothing (see above) should be proffered. Small doses of creams, applied when the itching is intense, containing 1 per cent hydrocortisone along with an antibiotic such as neomycin (to prevent secondary infection following scratching) are often very helpful. As pruritus seems to be particularly bad in bed at night, a mild sedative may aid sleep.
[C:655; H:248; J:562]

639   This is a skin condition in which there are a variety of epithelial changes associated with chronic pruritus. They may be hypotrophic, hypertrophic or dysplastic.
[C:658; E:159; G:109; J:329]

640   These are areas of hypertrophic squamous epithelium previously known as leucoplakia. There may be associated areas of dysplasia. Biopsy is generally advisable. In about 10 per cent of cases of dysplasia, frank malignant change may intervene.
[C:660; E:159; G:111; H:244; J:329]

641   This usually comes to the attention of the gynaecologist because of long standing pruritus. The skin is most often discoloured (red or white). Multiple biopsies are necessary to exclude any areas of frank malignancy and simple vulvectomy is the treatment of choice once the diagnosis has been confirmed.
[C:660; E:164]

642   The elderly. It is an uncommon condition in the premenopausal woman.
[E:167; H:254]

643   In the majority of cases, the patient complains of a sore or ulcer that fails to heal, or a persistent lump. Often the condition is bilateral (the so-called kissing ulcer).
[C:661; E:164; H:256]

644   No. The primary treatment is always surgical. Radical vulvectomy with localised lymphadenectomy should be attempted if the general condition of the patient permits. Local radiotherapy is contraindicated because the vulval area is difficult to keep dry and massive skin sloughing may ensue. In the very debilitated, simple excision under local or regional block should be carried out.
[C:682; H:258]

645   Pregnancy, when they may increase in size and profusion very rapidly, and profuse trichomonal infections.
[C:674; E:168; G:107; J:369]

646   The skin around the warts is covered with a protective layer of paraffin wax or similar substance and the warts painted with a 25 per cent solution of podophyllin in tincture of benzoin. This is removed by bathing after 6 hours and the procedure repeated on alternate days until the warts have disappeared.

Crystals of trichloracetic acid can be used in a similar way. In pregnancy podophyllin is contraindicated and if the warts are profuse, they are best removed by electocautery under general anaesthesia. Cryocautery is sometimes advocated but is very much less effective.
[C:675; E:168; J:370]

647   Fibromata and lipomata are common as are infected hair follicles and sebaceous cysts. Pilonidal sinus may occur in the clitoral area. Hydradenomata, melanoma, haemangioma and endometrioma have all been reported.
[C:674; H:248]

648   It is a reddened area involving the posterior urethral margin and probably represents a degree of urethral prolapse. The term was originally used to describe the polypoid type which is a deep red and exquisitely tender to touch, giving rise to dysuria and sometimes bleeding. Angiomatous and granulomatous variations are now described and, in their chronic state, are usually asymptomatic. Treatment for all types is diathermy excision.
[C:688; H:260; J:381]

649   This is a mucus retention cyst caused by the blockage of the duct leading from Bartholin's gland. The cyst may enlarge and become infected.
[C:687; H:230]

650   Marsupialisation of the cyst. A cruciate incision is made into it close to the hymeneal ring and the four flaps of skin formed are excised leaving a large stoma for drainage. The cyst wall is stitched to the skin edge. In time the cyst and stoma shrink leaving some functional gland behind.

651   It may rupture spontaneously, subside or become infected. In the latter case, a large abscess may form which is acutely uncomfortable. Treatment should always be surgical (drainage and marsupialisation). If treated with antibiotics and rest, recurrence is most probable.
[E:168]

652   These are shallow, red, intensely painful ulcers

caused by the herpes simplex type II virus. They may occur cyclically or at any time. Treatment is symptomatic, aimed at relieving the pain with local analgesia and preventing secondary infection. Application of idoxuridine has been advocated but does not seem to be any more efficacious. It is imperative that cervical herpetic lesions are looked for and long term cytology carried out on affected patients because of the risk of cervical intra-epithelial neoplasia.
[C:657; E:167; H:242]

H Diseases of the vagina

653 The glycogen found in the squamous cells of the vaginal epithelium is converted into lactic acid by Döderlein's bacilli (lactobacilli) which maintain the pH at about 4.
[E:170]

654 It is a white, non-offensive vaginal discharge made up of desquamated epithelial cells, non-pathogenic bacteria, vaginal transudate and cervical mucus. It is not pathological and does not require treatment.
[E:170; G:116; H:262]

655 The discharge is thick, white and non-offensive and leads to intense pruritus. Vaginal examination will reveal thick plaques likened to cottage cheese which, when removed, leave a reddened inflamed area of vagina. Confirmation of the diagnosis is made by vaginal swab and subsequent culture.
[E:172; G:119; H:266; J:312]

656 Nystatin pessaries are effective in over 90 per cent of patients if used daily for 7 days. However, they are messy, stain the underwear yellow and patient compliance is poor. More recent drugs such as clotrimazole, econazole and miconazole are equally as effective, needed for shorter duration and are less messy. It is most important that the partner of the patient is treated with a suitable cream containing the drug of choice, particularly if he has not been circumcised. For chronic sufferers long term treatment for 6 weeks to 3 months

may be necessary. Ketoconazole, which is taken orally, is probably the drug of choice as it is likely to remove reservoirs of infection in the alimentary tract.
[E:173; G:119]

657 The organism may exist in the vagina of some women without any symptoms and is only discovered on routine cervical screening. However, in those with symptoms, there is a profuse, greenish watery discharge which is slightly frothy. It has a very characteristic odour which is often what brings the patient to the doctor. Confirmation of the diagnosis can be made by mixing a drop of the discharge with a drop of saline on a slide and examining it microscopically at once. The motile flagellates will be visible in profusion.
[E:172; G:119; H:264]

658 Oral metronidazole 200 mg three times a day for one week will eradicate the organism in 98 per cent of patients. The male partner must be treated at the same time. Patients must be warned that the drug may react unfavourably with alcohol leading to severe nausea or vomiting.
[E:172; G:119; H:264; J:309]

659 Cysts of the mesonephric duct (Gärtner's) occur anterolaterally and are soft and asymptomatic and usually found in the upper vagina. Simple marsupialisation is all that is necessary. Suburethral cysts in Skene's ducts may give rise to urinary symptoms of frequency and dysuria. Excision is necessary.

Adenosis and adenocarcinoma are very rare but much publicity has been given to a number of cases, mainly in the USA, where the mothers of patients were treated early in pregnancy with diethyl stilboestrol. Subsequently, a very small percentage of the daughters of the successful pregnancies developed the condition in adolescence. The recommended treatment has been radical surgery. Other causes of carcinoma are (a) secondary, either by spread or metastases from the cervix, endometrium and more rarely ovary and kidney, and (b) primary squamous cell, the latter very occasionally arising in a chronic ulcer caused by long term use of a ring pessary.
[C:689; H:271]

660   The prepubertal vagina lacks the acidity of the adult and is quickly colonised by non-pathogenic bacteria. Inflammation of the vulva and vagina can lead to swelling, irritation, discharge and in the very young, fusion of the labia minora. The cause, in the majority of cases, is non-specific but *E. Coli, N. gonorrhoeae*, fungal or protozoal infections may occur. The introduction of foreign bodies by the child is often feared by the mother and can be excluded by gentle rectal examination or, very rarely, examination under anaesthesia. In general, cleanliness and daily washing with mild soap. careful drying and powdering of the vulva and the avoidance of nylon underwear usually suffices. If the labia are fused they can usually be separated digitally and oestrogen cream applied on alternate days for two weeks. Where a specific cause is found, specific therapy is indicated.
[E:271; G:117; I:307]

661   The skin of the postmenopausal vagina is thin and atrophic. The pH is much higher than that in the reproductive years because of the absence of lactobacilli and infection with bowel bacteria may occur. On examination, the walls of the vagina appear red with tiny vessels close to the suface which bleed easily with minimal trauma. Treatment is with local oestrogen creams or pessaries but systemic oestrogens may be used. If bleeding is the presenting symptom, then curettage must also be undertaken to exclude an intrauterine pathology.
[G:120; H:270; J:308]

I   Diseases of the cervix

662   Mucus secreted by the columnar epithelial cells or glands of the cervix reaches the surface by means of ducts. At various stages of a woman's life squamous metaplasia take place—that is, the columnar epithelium becomes covered by squamous epithelium and the ducts and mucus secreting glands become buried. Mucus continues to be secreted and retention cysts form. These are known as Nabothian follicles. They do not cause symptoms and are of little significance.
[E:177; J:316]

663   Cervical polyp.
      [H:293]

664   Cervical polyps are nodular or pedunculated growths from the endocervix. Occasionally polypoidal fibroids may also present at the cervical os. The main symptoms are vaginal discharge which may be bloodstained if the polyp is ulcerated. Contact bleeding may also occur and occasionally the polyp may be large enough for the patient to be aware of its presence in the vagina or at the introitus. Treatment is avulsion of the polyp and cautery to the polyp base. Dilatation of the cervix and curettage should be carried out at the same time to remove any other polyps that may be present and to rule out other causes of symptoms especially carcinoma.
      [H:293]

665   It is a zone of columnar epithelium visible on the vaginal portion of the cervix and the term cervical erosion is misleading. Eversion of the columnar epithelium on to the ectocervix often gives the cervix a reddened or raw appearance and this 'ectropion' is often incorrectly termed a cervical erosion. It occurs as a physiological process in fetal development, at puberty and in pregnancy and seldom gives rise to symptoms.
      [C:165; G:122]

666   A patient with a cervical erosion is very often asymptomatic. On occasions, however, the patient complains of a vaginal discharge produced by the mucus-secreting columnar cells. This can become offensive if the epithelium becomes abraded and infected, resulting in cervicitis. Staining or bleeding can sometimes occur following intercourse or when taking a cervical smear.
      [E:177; G:126]

667   The findings of a cervical erosion on gynaecological examination require a cervical smear to be taken. If this is normal, further treatment depends on the symptoms. If there are no symptoms no treatment is necessary. If discharge is troublesome, cautery to the cervix is often helpful.

668   He was an American anatomist who in 1943

stated that the cervix was an accessible area of the female body where cancerous changes in the cells could be easily sampled, stained and identified.

669 All patients who are or have been sexually active should have a smear. From the teens to 35 years, smears should be carried out every 3–5 years and from 35 to 60 every 3 years. However, the frequency may be increased at the discretion of the physician, dependent upon the presence of gynaecological disease, method of contraception and parity of the patient.

670 A study of single cells scraped from the epithelial surface of the cervix. Exfoliated cells from premalignant or malignant sites show variations in size and shape. An increase in the nucleocytoplasmic ratio is seen as well as intense nuclear staining. Experienced cytologists are able to differentiate from mildly abnormal forms of dyskaryosis to carcinoma *in situ*. Invasive lesions are also identifiable.
[H:317; J:490]

671 Dyskaryosis is a term used to describe abnormal appearances of exfoliated squamous cells.

672 Carcinoma *in situ* describes an epithelium in which there is full thickness loss of cell differentiation. The squamous cells varying in shape and size with an increased nucleocytoplasmic ratio with frequent bizarre mitotic figures. Dysplasia is the histological description of a lesion in which some degree of differentation of the epithelium may have been retained.
[C:705; H:305]

673 This varies from one country to another but five grades are recognised, namely: normal, mild dyskaryosis, moderate dyskaryosis, severe dyskaryosis, carcinoma *in situ*.
[C:707; E:181]

674 The term cervical intraepithelial neoplasia (CIN) is used to emphasise the continuum of the disease from mild to severe dysplasia and carcinoma *in situ*. CIN I corresponds to mild

dysplasia. CIN II corresponds to moderate dysplasia. CIN III corresponds to severe dysplasia and carcinoma *in situ*. There is no biological difference between the last two lesions.

675   There are degrees of dysplasia (mild, moderate and severe) and the most mild are probably reversible and easily regress. Severe dysplasia and carcinoma *in situ* may progress to invasive cancer in between 10 and 30 per cent of patients.
[C:713; H:307]

676   There is now convincing evidence notably from British Columbia and Aberdeen that with almost complete population cover, the incidence of invasive cancer can be markedly reduced as a result of mass cervical screening programmes.
[C:712; H:320]

677   The colposcope is an optical instrument providing an illuminated magnified view of the uterine cervix. It allows the exact site and extent of premalignant lesions to be defined and biopsies may be easily performed giving a 96 per cent accuracy when compared to eventual histology from operative specimens. Cervical smears can indicate an abnormality of the cervix. Colposcopy can pinpoint the exact spot or area. This has important bearing on subsequent treatment.
[C:707; H:321]

678   The transformation zone is an area of columnar epithelium which has undergone squamous metaplasia. It always lies between native squamous epithelium and native columnar epithelium.
[C:708]

679   It is an area where squamous metaplasia has taken place in an atypical fashion and represents the area in which squamous carcinoma of the cervix arises.
[C:708]

680   Any signs of infection should be treated and the smear should be repeated. All patients with positive smears and those with persistent

dyskaryosis should be referred to the gynaecological department and ideally a colposcopic examination carried out.
[E:187]

681   (a) Cone biopsy.
      (b) Conservative   methods: cryosurgery; electrocautery; carbon dioxide laser.
      (c) Total abdominal hysterectomy.
      [H:328]

682   Any patient with a positive cervical smear necessitates the gynaecologist to first rule out the presence of obvious invasive cancer. If colposcopy is unavailable or unsatisfactory (as it is in 10 per cent of patients where the lesion extends into the endocervical canal so obscuring the upper limits of the disease), a cone biopsy must be carried out. This provides adequate tissue for diagnosis and is also adequate treatment for the majority of premalignant lesions.
      [H:326]

683   It requires a general anaesthetic. There are risks of both immediate and secondary haemorrhage. There is significant impairment of fertility in subsequent pregnancies—notably an increased incidence of premature labour and low birth weight babies. The caesarean section rate also seems to be higher.
      [C:710]

684   The main indication is for those patients with coexistent gynaecological disease, notably fibroids or menstrual disturbances, or those who have completed their family. In approximately 4 per cent of cases, the lesion extends onto the vaginal fornices which may be recognised colposcopically. This allows those cases to be treated by hysterectomy with a cuff of vagina whilst the other 96 per cent can be treated by simple hysterectomy.
      [C:710; H:328]

685   With the advent of mass cervical screening more women under the age of 35 are being found who require treatment. Many of these have yet to start or complete their families and hysterectomy would be too drastic a treatment. Cone biopsy may also impair future fertility

and for these reasons more conservative measures have been adopted.

686   It is successful, with 95 per cent cure rates already reported. It can be done as an out-patient procedure without anaesthesia. It is relatively painless and free from side effects. Directed through a colposcope it allows very precise vaporisation of the diseased area and transformation zone with little damage to surrounding tissue. It allows for satisfactory follow-up by cervical cytology. It reduces the need for cone biopsy by up to 80 per cent. It seems likely that future fertility is not impaired.

687   Punch biopsy under colposcopic control is the treatment of choice. Cone biopsy is not recommended because of the risk of causing abortion (20 per cent) and the risk of severe haemorrhage (30 per cent). For frankly invasive lesions, the pregnancy should be terminated if before 30 weeks' gestation and the patient then treated by radiotherapy or Wertheim's hysterectomy 2 weeks later. If the pregnancy is advanced to 30 weeks or more, delivery should be delayed to the 34th week and then caesarean section employed.

688   None whatsoever. Pregnancy does not increase the likelihood of the lesion becoming invasive.

689   No. Vaginal delivery will not increase the likelihood of the disease spreading or becoming invasive. (Vaginal delivery in patients with invasive carcinoma of the cervix does increase the risk of spread and delivery should be by classical caesarean section.)

690   The commonest malignant tumour of the genital tract is carcinoma of the cervix.
      [E:189]

691   The aetiology of carcinoma of the cervix has still to be finally elucidated but the following factors are relevant:
      (a) age at first coitus and promiscuity—in one survey, over half the patients with cancer of the cervix had intercourse before the age

of 17. Cervical cancer is also more prevalent in prostitutes.

(b) social status—carcinoma of the cervix is more prevalent in the lower socioeconomic groups.

(c) race—for some reason Jewesses are at a very low risk of developing carcinoma of the cervix.

(d) carcinogens—a higher incidence of carcinoma of the cervix is found in patients with herpes simplex virus (type II).

[C:705; H:297]

692 There are two histological types of cervical carcinoma. The vast majority, 95 per cent, arise from the squamous epithelium in the transformation zone—squamous cell carcinoma (epidermoid carcinoma). The remaining group adenocarcinoma—accounts for 5 per cent of cases and arise from the endocervical columnar cells. If carcinoma of the cervix presents under the age of 20 years, it is invariably an adenocarcinoma.
[E:190]

693 The presentation of carcinoma of the cervix is variable. In the early stages of the disease there are no symptoms. In the later stages irregular and postcoital bleeding and offensive vaginal discharge are characteristic. Pain is an even later symptom as is urinary incontinence, weight loss and malaise.
[C:714; E:192; G:186; H:316; J:398]

694 Carcinoma of the cervix spreads by the following routes:
(a) direct spread—to related organs, upwards to involve the uterus or downwards to involve the vagina eventually involving bladder and rectum. Lateral spread also occurs to the pelvic side wall where obstruction of the ureter can occur.

(b) lymphatic spread—usually follows but may precede direct spread. The cervix has a rich lymphatic supply and there is usually early lymphatic involvement, usually of the iliac and obturator nodes.
[E:191]

695 The clinical staging of cervical carcinoma is as follows:

Stage 0— preinvasive carcinoma or carcinoma *in situ*.

Stage I— carcinoma confined to the cervix (extension to the corpus is disregarded).

Ia— preclinical invasive carcinoma which cannot be diagnosed with the naked eye.

Ib— all other cases of Stage I.

Stage II— the carcinoma extends beyond the cervix but has not extended to the pelvic wall. The carcinoma involves the vagina but not the lower third.

IIa— no obvious parametrial involvement.

IIb— obvious parametrial involvement.

Stage III— the carcinoma has extended onto the pelvic wall. On rectal examination there is no cancer-free space between the tumour and the pelvic wall. The tumour involves the lower third of the vagina.

Presence of hydronephrosis of non-functioning kidney.

IIIa— no extension on to the pelvic wall.

IIIb— extension on to the pelvic wall.

Stage IV — the carcinoma has extended beyond the true pelvis or has involved the mucosa of the bladder or the rectum. The presence of bullous oedema is not sufficient evidence to classify a case of Stage IV.

[C:716; E:192; G:188; H:328; J:403]

696 There has been much debate about the treatment of carcinoma of the cervix which has led, regrettably, to rigid attitudes. Initially, radical surgery with pelvic lymphadenectomy, as described by Wertheim, was the only available method that had some measure of success. Later radiotherapy was introduced and nowadays it is the basis of treatment, surgery with or without radiotherapy being used only for carefully selected cases.
[C:718; H:331]

697 The advantages of surgical treatment of carcinoma of the cervix are that the primary growth and drainage area are removed. Also in

expert hands the results are as good and in some cases slightly better than results achieved by radiotherapy and any pelvic inflammation can be dealt with at the time of operation. For some patients surgery is preferable to radiotherapy, particularly in the young with Stage I or IIa disease, when the ovaries can be conserved. Surgery is the only treatment of some radioresistant growths.
[E:193]

698   The disadvantages of surgical treatment of carcinoma of the cervix are:
   (a) The mortality rate is approximately 1–2 per cent.
   (b) The tumour must be operable and not fixed to pelvic wall.
   (c) The patient must be a good surgical candidate and not grossly obese.
   (d) Ureteric fistula are likely to develop, even in the most skilled hands in 1–5 per cent of cases.
   (e) It requires a surgeon skilled at radical pelvic surgery.

J   Diseases of the uterus

699   It is a localised overgrowth of the endometrium and may occur premenopausally or postmenopausally. It is often associated with endometrial hyperplasia and in these cases the patients may have dysfunctional uterine bleeding. Most likely, however, the patient will present with intermenstrual or postmenopausal bleeding. Although they must never be considered premalignant, a relationship with the subsequent development of adenocarcinoma has been noted.
[C:697; E:195; G:175; H:387; J:412]

700   Cystic glandular hyperplasia and adenomatous (atypical) hyperplasia. Both may occur at either end of reproductive life as a result of unopposed oestrogen activity, and both give rise to dysfunctional uterine bleeding. Adenomatous hyperplasia is considered to be a premalignant (carcinoma *in situ*) condition.
[E:196; G:254; H:377; J:345]

701   This depends upon her age, her desire to retain

her reproductive capabilities and, in the case of adenomatous hyperplasia, the degree of atypia present. In the younger woman, cyclical progestogens over many months, or continuous use over a number of weeks usually effects a cure. At the climaceteric, gestagens are usually preferred for the treatment of cystic hyperplasia, but when atypia exists, hysterectomy is the treatment of choice.
[E:196; H:384; J:348]

702 A fibromyoma or leiomyoma. It can occur anywhere along the Müllerian duct but is most commonly associated with the myometrium. It is the most common tumour of the human body and occurs in one in five of all women at death. The tumour consists of smooth muscle bundles and has a characteristic whorled appearance. The size may vary from microscopic to huge. They are more commonly seen in nulliparous women or women of low parity and black women are far more prone to the condition.
[C:698; E:205; G:157; H:427; J:413]

703 In most cases they are contained within the myometrium (intramural), but they can occur projecting from the peritoneal surface of the uterus (subserous), or distort the uterine cavity (submucous). Subserous fibroids may become pedunculated and submucous fibroids polypoidal. They may also be found in the cervix, or broad ligament. Fibroids found attached to other structures such as the omentum are pedunculated fibroids that have gained a secondary blood supply from the structure and become detached from the uterus.
[C:698; E:206; G:158; H:427; J:415]

704 The tumour is relatively avascular, being supplied by blood from its pseudocapsule of compressed endometrium. This commonly leads to degenerative changes which can be:
    (a) hyaline. Large areas of hyaline change may become liquefied leading to
    (b) cystic changes.
    (c) calcified, which are more common in pedunculated fibroids and are seen in older women. These become what were known as 'womb-stones.'

(d) infective. This is unusual except when fibroids become attached to bowel or areas of pelvic infection.

(e) red degeneration. This is more commonly seen in pregnancy but can occur at other times. There is thrombosis in peripheral veins leading to engorgement and rupture of capillary plexi. The cut surface is likened to raw beef.

(f) sarcomatous. This is extremely rare occurring in less than one-half per cent of patients.

[C:699; E:207; G:162; H:434; J:426]

705   This depends upon the size and position of the myoma. The most common symptom is an increase in menstrual loss. This may be due to the increased vascularity of the uterus or distortion and enlargement of the cavity. The tumour may give rise to no symptoms at all until it fills the pelvis and becomes palpable abdominally. Pressure on the bladder may give rise to frequency and occasionally stress incontinence. Backache is common but constipation is not related to fibroids. A fibroid polyp may give rise to very acute colicky dysmenorrhoea and, if necrosis of the apex occurs, intermenstrual bleeding and discharge. Unless the fibroids distort the uterine cavity or occlude both tubes, they are not a cause of infertility, but they are, of course, much more common in the nulliparous patient and the two are therefore associated by chance. Rarely, a fibroid may be the cause of acute retroversion and retention of urine in the same manner as an impacted retroverted gravid uterus. The effect of fibroids in pregnancy is discussed elsewhere.

[C:700; E:207; G:168; H:437; J:415]

706   There is a definite place for conservative management when fibroids are asymptomatic. Because of their tendency to grow in the reproductive years they should be reviewed annually and surgery contemplated when symptoms occur. If menorrhagia is present and the fibroids distort the uterine cavity, either removal of the fibroids (myomectomy) or removal of the uterus (hysterectomy) must be considered. The decision as to which operation

is carried out depends upon the patient's age and her desire or otherwise, to retain her reproductive capacity. It is normal to recommend surgery to patients in whom uterine enlargement exceeds the equivalent of a 14 week pregnancy because pressure symptoms are common. Myomectomy must never be attempted if the patient is pregnant.
[C:701; E:208; G:172; H:440; J:420]

707 The differential diagnosis lies between uterine fibroids, and an ovarian cyst (and occasionally, a full bladder!). On bimanual examination, the cervix will move if the uterus is pushed from side to side if fibroids are present. If a cyst exists, the uterus should be felt, usually anteriorly, as a separate structure. However, the distinction is often much more difficult than it sounds. Ultrasonic examination is usually able to clarify the situation. In either case laparotomy is essential and the appropriate action taken.
[G:171; J:474]

708 Adenocarcinoma of the endometrium. It occurs almost as commonly as carcinoma of the cervix but is usually detected at a much earlier stage and therefore success rates are considerably better.
[E:197; G:194; H:391]

709 It is predominantly a disease of the postmenopausal woman, the peak age incidence being between 55 and 60, although about 20 per cent of cases are diagnosed prior to the menopause. The patients are usually overweight, of low or nil parity, have a late menopause and may show evidence of altered carbohydrate metabolism. Obese women have higher circulating oestrogen levels and it is unopposed oestrogen secretion that is thought to be the cause of atypical changes in the endometrium. The prognosis depends upon the degree of differentiation of the tumour.
[C:731; E:198; G:194; H:391; J:429]

710 In almost all cases, the initial symptom is postmenopausal bleeding (or irregular bleeding at the perimenopausal stage). As has been stated earlier, any postmenopausal woman

with bleeding from the vagina must have a diagnostic curettage to exclude an intrauterine malignancy.
[C:736; E:202; G:196; H:410]

711   Stage   I—the growth is confined to the corpus uteri.

Stage   II—the growth involves the corpus and the cervix.

Stage III—the growth extends beyond the uterus but not outside the true pelvis.

Stage IV—the growth extends beyond the true pelvis or involves the mucosa of the bladder or rectum.

Stage I growths are further subdivided depending upon whether the length of the uterine cavity is more than 8 cm, or 8 cm and less. As already stated, the degree of differentiation is of considerable importance.

Three-quarters of patients in whom the diagnosis is made, fall within the Stage I category.
[C:735; E:203; G:197; H:414]

712   The treatment of Stage I disease is essentially one of surgery—bilateral oophorectomy and total hysterectomy. Radiotherapy is usually given postoperatively if penetration of the growth exceeds one-third of the myometrium or if the growth is undifferentiated. Some centres still prefer to use radiotherapy preoperatively but this does mean a proportion of patients are treated unnecessarily. There is rapidly growing evidence that high dose gestagen therapy given preoperatively and continued for at least 3 months after surgery, improves survival rates.
[C:737; E:203; G:197; H:416; J:434]

713   In Stage II, the cervix is involved and therefore different lymphatics to those that drain the corpus. Radical surgery (Wertheim hysterectomy) should be attempted if the patient's size and condition permits but radiotherapy is the main line of treatment. In Stages III and IV, localised radiotherapy is of some use and high dose progestogen therapy may cause remarkable remissions in the disease, particularly in the very old.
[C:739; H:422; J:435]

714   This depends upon the staging and differenti-
       ation of the growth. In Stage I, 5-year survival
       of about 80 per cent can be expected. In Stages
       II, III, and IV, the figures are approximately 45
       per cent, 30 per cent and 15 per cent respect-
       ively.
       [C:739; G:422]

K   Diseases of the fallopian tubes

715   There are three routes of spread, by ascending
       infection via the vagina, cervix and uterus; by
       spread from the pelvic peritoneum; and by
       haematogenous spread (the latter is nearly
       always tuberculous). The condition may be
       acute, subacute or chronic.
       [C:526; E:148; G:132; H:462]

716   In the past, infection with *Neisseria gonorrhoeae*
       was believed to account for 60–70 per cent of
       cases, although bacteriological confirmation
       was only available in a proportion of these. It is
       now known that infection with *Chlamydia*, *Bac-
       teroides* and Gram-negative streptococci
       account for many cases. The patient presents
       with a high temperature, 39 °C or more (102 °F)
       and the pulse is rapid. There is acute lower
       abdominal tenderness with guarding and
       rigidity. There is often vomiting and the
       patient may have a violent headache. She may
       complain of an offensive vaginal discharge,
       often bloodstained and dysuria and frequency
       of micturition. Vaginal examination reveals
       marked tenderness especially on moving the
       cervix and there may be bilateral adnexal
       swelling. The white cell count is usually in
       excess of 15 000/mm^3 and the erythrocyte sedi-
       mentation rate very raised.
       [C:527; E:148; G:135; H:467; J:322]

717   There is acute inflammation of the tubes with
       infiltration by polymorphonuclear cells of the
       muscularis. The endosalpinx is only minimally
       involved at first. If no treatment is commenced
       the ovaries may become involved leading to a
       tubo-ovarian abscess or, at a later stage, a
       pelvic abscess. The fimbriae may become
       sealed and further pus formation cause a
       pyosalpinx. If treatment is available many of

these changes will be halted but the long term sequelae of the infection will include pelvic adhesions, fimbrial occlusion, ovarian adhesions, hydrosalpinx and damage to the endosalpinx. The severity of the changes will depend upon the infecting organism and the type and timing of treatment.
[C:526; H:464; J:320]

718 (a) Acute appendicitis. The fever is usually lower, the white cell count is unreliable, headache is not usually a feature and classically the pain starts periumbilically and moves to the right lower quadrant.
 (b) Tubal pregnancy. Fever is not common and amenorrhoea is usually a feature. There is no leucocytosis.
 (c) Ovarian cyst undergoing torsion or rupture. Pain is very acute and colicky if torsion is occurring. Vomiting is common. There is usually no fever and the symptoms tend to be unilateral.
 (d) Acute pyelitis. There is fever and pain but the leucocytosis is lower than with salpingitis and the urine is infected. If there is any doubt about the diagnosis, laparoscopy must be undertaken.
[C:527; E:152; G:136; H:469; J:323]

719 Prior to commencement of therapy, swabs should be taken from urethra, cervix and rectum. Treatment with a broad spectrum antibiotic such as ampicillin may be very effective but resistance to the penicillins is increasing. Probenecid given in conjunction with ampicillin will maintain the blood levels. Concurrent treatment with metronidazole is generally given to combat *Bacteroides* infection. In the acutely ill patient, gentamicin given intravenously is useful. In the shocked patient, prompt resuscitation is important, particular attention being paid to fluid and electrolyte balance. In postabortal or puerperal patients, endometrial curettage should be performed after resuscitation has been carried out and antibiotic therapy been commenced. Otherwise there is seldom a need for surgical intervention except where the diagnosis is in doubt (see above). Antibiotic therapy should be continued for 10–14 days.
[C:527; E:152; G:137; H:472]

720 *E. coli*, streptococci, staphylococci, *Bacteroides* are the most common. The clostridii and tetanus bacteria tend to lead to generalised septicaemia rather than salpingitis.
[E:151; J:319]

721 It is an important cause of dysmenorrhoea, dyspareunia, menorrhagia and pelvic pain. It often follows inadequate treatment of the acute phase of the disease and may present one of the most trying of problems for the gynaecologist. Chronic backache and Mittelschmerz often occur and many have a copious purulent discharge. However, others may be asymptomatic and the condition only discovered during investigation of subfertility.
[C:530; E:153; G:136; H:478; J:323]

722 There is usually tenderness in one or both iliac fossae and occasionally a pelvic swelling may be palpated. On vaginal examination, the uterus is often fixed and retroverted (by pelvic adhesions) and there is tenderness and adnexal thickening. The clinical picture is not complete until laparoscopy or laparotomy is undertaken.
[C:530; E:154; G:136; H:478]

723 This depends upon the patient's age, parity and symptoms. Conservative management is usually attempted in the young and is mainly long term antibiotic therapy. The results are disappointing. Treatment with pelvic short-wave diathermy was popular but there is little or no evidence that it helps and may indeed exacerbate symptoms. Surgery should be radical, except in cases where subfertility is a problem and there is a possibility of tubal surgery. In other cases, the uterus, tubes and often the ovaries must be removed especially if there is a deterioration in the health of the patient, there is a persistence in pelvic pain or size of the pelvic masses, menorrhagia becomes intolerable or there are repeated acute exacerbations of the disease.
[C:531; E:154; G:138; H:478; J:324]

724 Endometriosis. Very occasionally fibroids or ovarian cysts may present with a similar picture.
[C:530; G:137]

725 In the past, the incidence of the disease has been reported as being between 2 and 5 per cent in the UK. However, since the introduction of drug therapy the incidence has declined and is below 1 per cent amongst the indigenous population. In areas with a high immigrant population, especially Asians, tuberculosis still represents an important cause of infertility. The disease is almost always secondary to a primary lesion elsewhere in the body and spread is usually haematogenous from a pulmonary lesion.
[C:532; E:155; G:139; H:484]

726 In many cases the patients are asymptomatic except for involuntary subfertility. At the other extreme there may be evidence of pelvic masses and the patient has fever, night sweats, loss of weight and general malaise. Menstrual irregularity is common and in cases where the endometrium is destroyed, amenorrhoea may be a presenting symptom. Very rarely it may cause postmenopausal bleeding.
[C:533; E:155; G:141; H:488; J:295]

727 The condition usually involves both tubes which become thickened and rigid. Tubercles may be noted on their surface. Occasionally a pyosalpinx may develop. Caseation may be noted on microscopy as is the classical infiltration with giant and epithelioid cells. The infecting organism is almost always the human *Mycobacterium tuberculosis* (as distinct from the bovine form). The endometrium is commonly involved.
[C:432; E:155; G:139; H:484; J:294]

728 Premenstrual curettage is essential. The curettings are examined for the presence of tubercles and, after Ziehl–Neelson staining, for evidence of *Mycobacterium tuberculosis*. When the condition is suspected, culture and sensitivity tests are carried out, as is inoculation of endometrial tissue into a guinea-pig. Salpingography may be employed but runs the risk of causing a 'flare-up.' (This is less likely with modern water soluble radio-opaque dyes.) The classical findings are narrow rigid 'pipe-stem' tubes with evidence of crypts and sinuses, clubbing of the ampulla and calcification in tubes or ovaries. Laparoscopy may show evidence of tubercles

which can be biopsied for microscopic examination. The Mantoux intradermal test will be strongly positive in affected patients.
[C:533; E:156; G:141; H:489; J:297]

729   Chemotherapy must be started even before bacteriological confirmation. Various drugs or combinations of drugs are used and treatment should be carried out in conjunction with a chest physician. Streptomycin with isoniazid for 3 months followed by isoniazid and para-aminosalicylic acid for 18 months has been standard treatment for many years. Currently rifampicin and isoniazid is employed with the addition of ethambutol for the first 9–12 weeks. Surgery may be necessary in some patients, particularly those who have finished reproducing and who have gynaecological problems such as severe menstrual problems or the persistence of pelvic masses. Hysterectomy and bilateral salpingo-oophorectomy should be carried out and drug therapy continued as outlined above.
[C:533; E:156; G:142; H:491; J:298]

730   It is an embryological remnant of the upper end of the Müllerian duct which is represented by an asymptomatic small cyst attached to one of the tubal fimbria.
[G:84; H:501; J:129]

731   This is an exceedingly rare adenocarcinoma presenting usually as a copious serosanguinous discharge. A palpable mass is found in two-thirds of cases. Presentation is late for the same reasons as with ovarian cancer and the prognosis is poor.
[C:742; G:201; H:496; J:441]

L   Diseases of the ovaries

732   The surface covering is known as the germinal, serosal, coelomic or Müllerian epithelium. It was originally thought that the epithelium gave rise to the germ cells, hence the erroneous but commonly used term, germinal epithelium. It is, in fact, modified peritoneum of Müllerian (and therefore coelomic) origin. The

other two main components are the germ cells and medullary or mesenchymal elements.

733 These functional cysts of the ovaries are either of follicular or luteal origin. They may arise as an imbalance of pituitary gonadotrophin secretion or may result from ovarian stimulation with clomiphene citrate or systemic gonadotrophin therapy. They are seldom large, usually symptomless and, most often, disappear spontaneously.
[E:246; G:207; H:509]

734 Cysts may undergo torsion, rupture or haemorrhage. Occasionally they can become infected. They may give rise to constant, intermittent or recurring pain. Functional cysts may cause menstrual abnormalities. When very large, frequency of micturition may occur and uterovaginal prolapse may be exacerbated. Until removed, a diagnosis of malignancy cannot be excluded especially in patients over the age of 35.
[C:745; E:244; G:227; H:511; J:448]

735 Pregnancy; a full bladder; fibroids, particularly a large solitary myoma undergoing cystic degeneration; obesity, pseudocyesis; ascites.
[C:747; E:243; G:229]

736 Hydrosalpinx or pyosalpinx; fimbrial cysts; myomata, particularly pedunculated ones; retroverted pregnant uterus; tubal pregnancy; full bladder; faeces in the small or large bowel.
[E:243; G:229]

737 First, empty the bladder, If you suspect that the bladder is full, even after voiding, catheterisation should be undertaken. On bimanual examination, the uterus should be felt as a separate structure to a cystic ovary and should move independently to the tumour. However, a soft pregnant uterus can cause confusion. Ultrasonic examination is very useful in cases where there is doubt and, for small pelvic tumours, laparoscopy may be invaluable.
[C:229; G:229]

738 The ovary is a very mobile structure lying in

the pelvis. Considerable enlargement can occur without causing any symptoms, and by the time symptoms of abdominal distension, anorexia, loss of weight and general debility are noted, the disease has reached a very late stage.
[C:747; E:251]

739　(a) Epithelial tumours (coelomic, germinal)—serous, mucinous, endometroid, mesonephroid, Brenner, mixed.
　　(b) Sex cord (mesenchymal or gonadal) tumours—granulosa (theca group), Sertoli (Leydig group), mixed (gynandroblastoma), indeterminate.
　　(c) Lipid (lipoid) cell tumours.
　　(d) Germ cell tumours—disgerminoma (seminoma), endodermal sinus tumour, embryonal carcinoma, choriocarcinoma, teratoma (dermoid cysts).
　　(e) Gonadoblastoma.
　　(f) Unclassified tumours.
　　(g) Secondary (metastatic tumours).
[E:246; G:206; H:507]

740　Serous cysts are most frequently found in the third to fifth decades of life. They may be very large but seldom attain the huge proportions of the mucinous variety. Serous cysts are much more likely to undergo malignant change (30 per cent compared to 5–10 per cent for the mucinous cyst). Mucinous cysts are multiloculated whereas serous cysts tend to contain only a few cavities. Papilliferous outgrowths may occur on the inner and outer surfaces of serous cysts giving an appearance of malignancy when they may, in fact, be benign. Mucinous cysts occasionally rupture, releasing their contents into the peritoneal cavity. Cells from the tumour implant on peritoneum and bowel and continue to form mucin, leading to a condition known as myxoma peritonei. This may cause massive adhesions and, although histologically benign, can lead to the death of the patient.
[C:752; E:247; G:209; H:517; J:457]

741　Treatment is dependent upon the age of the patient and extent of the disease. Oophorectomy is usually necessary and as the condition may be bilateral, both ovaries may have to be

sacrificed. In the younger woman, every attempt should be made to conserve ovarian tissue if the condition is benign but in the case of serous cysts, especially in women over the age of 40, bilateral oophorectomy is usually performed (with hysterectomy) because of the increased likelihood of malignant change.
[C:748; E:248; G:231; J:478]

742　These cysts are found usually in young women. They arise from germ cells and are therefore totipotential. However, ectodermal elements are usually predominant. They tend to be unilateral, about 10 cm in diameter and contain sebaceous material and hair. Teeth, bone and cartilage may occur and in rare instances gastric mucosa. Functional thyroid tissue very occasionally is present—the so-called struma ovarii.
[C:752; E:248; G:214; H:561; J:463]

743　This condition occurs when the predominant element in a malignant ovarian cyst appears closely related to endometrial carcinoma. In fact, in 20 per cent of cases there is an associated intrauterine pathology. It was initially thought that endometrioid adenocarcinoma arose from areas of ovarian endometriosis but this is thought to occur in only 5–10 per cent of cases, the remainder representing malignant change in Müllerian epithelium.
[C:759; H:530]

744　Stage　I—growth confined to the ovaries.
　　　Stage　II—growth involving ovaries with pelvic extension.
　　　Stage III—growth involving ovaries with intraperitoneal metastases beyond the confines of the pelvis.
　　　Stage IV—growth involving ovaries with distant metastases.
　　　Unfortunately at least 60 per cent of ovarian malignancies have spread beyond the ovaries when first discovered.
[C:750; G:223; H:516]

745　About 36–50 per cent are of serous origin and approximately 20 per cent for both endometrioid and mucinous tumours. 10–20 per cent are made up by the remaining types of epithelial tumours.
[C:237]

746   The first approach is always surgical. It is at operation that the diagnosis is usually made or confirmed. Modern opinion favours radical surgery in cases where the growth has spread beyond the ovaries. As much tumour is excised as possible, and this may include all the pelvic peritoneum. Both ovaries and uterus are removed. Omentectomy should be performed. Surgery must be followed by chemotherapy and radiotherapy, the usefulness of the latter being much debated at present. Chemotherapy has depended upon alkylating agents for many years but, recently, successes have been reported with *cis*-platinum and hexylmethylmelamine. Combination chemotherapy seems the most effective.
[C:749; E:251; G:231; H:544]

747   This is a particular variety of secondary ovarian tumour with a specific histological appearance. There is a mucoid accumulation in the cytoplasm of the cells displacing the flattened nucleus to one side and giving the appearance of a signet ring. The primary neoplasm is an adenocarcinoma arising, in most cases, from the gastrointestinal tract (usually the stomach).
[E:250; G:221; H:540; J:454]

748   This is an interesting but most unusual cause of hydrothorax and ascites. It is usually caused by a fibroma of the ovary and the supposed mechanism is peritoneal irritation by the hard mobile tumour. The origin of the hydrothorax is uncertain but lymphatics through the diaphragm seem the most likely route for the ascitic fluid. Removal of the tumour results in complete disappearance of the fluid.
[C:746; E:249; G:220; H:584; J:460]

M   Endometriosis

749   The term is applied to a condition where endometrium is found in situations other than the uterine cavity. If found in the myometrium, it is more commonly referred to as adenomyosis. Although histologically similar, the conditions probably result in different ways and usually occur in different types of patient.
[C:536; E:210; G:235; H:609; J:350]

750 Endometrial glands are present together with stroma, and there is evidence of recent or old bleeding. This contrasts with metastatic deposits of endometrial adenocarcinoma where stroma is not a feature and evidence of bleeding very uncommon.
[C:536; H:612; J:350]

751 This is a condition affecting older, multiparous women usually approaching the menopause. The principal feature is menorrhagia, but secondary dysmenorrhoea is common, as is dyspareunia. Pelvic examination reveals a tender bulky uterus.
[C:536; E:213; H:447; J:354]

752 Medical treatment is not common because the diagnosis can seldom be made until the uterus is removed. Hormonal therapy with progestogenic agents may be tried following curettage in those who wish to preserve their reproductive capabilities. Abdominal or vaginal hysterectomy is the preferred method of treatment. Except in the severely debilitated, there is no longer any place for treatment with radium.
[E:216; H:448; J:354]

753 Five theories are current.
(a) The implantation theory of Sampson suggests that menstrual blood containing endometrial tissue passes down the tubes and implants particularly on the ovaries and in the pouch of Douglas. Retrograde menstruation certainly occurs but the theory fails to explain deposits in sites which would not be reached by retrograde menstruation.
(b) Coelomic metaplasia has been propounded as a likely explanation. The peritoneum (and pleura) are all derived from the same coelomic tissue which also forms the Müllerian system. Immature groups of coelomic cells may undergo change into Müllerian epithelium under hormonal activity and this epithelium has the potential of forming endometrial epithelium.
(c) The imitative metaplasia theory is a combination of (a) and (b). It suggests that

endometrial cells shed by retrograde menstruation may stimulate metaplasia in susceptible epithelium. This seems the most likely cause of the condition.

(d) Lymphatic and haematogenous spread may account for the occasional distant deposits.

(e) Surgical implantation theory. This accounts for endometriotic deposits in abdominal wounds following hysterotomy.

[C:537; G:236; H:609; J:357]

754 The ovaries are the commonest site and chocolate cysts may develop. These contain old blood, but not all chocolate cysts are endometriotic in origin. The pelvic peritoneum, especially over the uterosacral ligaments, is also a common site. The deposits are present as either blue-black cystic lesions seldom more than 1 or 2 mm in diameter or as 'powder burn' points. More rarely, the deposits may be found in the large bowel causing fibrosis and stricture formation resembling malignant conditions of the bowel. Endometriosis may involve the bladder, vagina and cervix and is not uncommon in abdominal scars following hysterotomy. Paradoxically, it very rarely occurs after caesarean section.

[C:540; E:213; J:354]

755 The disease is much more common amongst white girls than amongst black and they are of the age group 25–35. The patients are usually nulliparous or of low parity. It is observed more in women of higher socioeconomic groups and seems to be increasing but the use of diagnostic laparoscopy has led to the recognition of the condition in many more women, many of whom are asymptomatic.

[J:352]

756 These are variable depending upon the site and extent of the disease. However, the size of the lesion may have little relationship to the severity of the symptoms. The typical symptoms are very similar to chronic pelvic infection and are comprised of pelvic pain (dysmenorrhoea, dyspareunia, Mittelschmerz), menorrhagia and infertility. Other symptoms include cyclical haematuria, bleeding per

rectum and very rarely cyclical haemoptysis. Intestinal obstruction can occur.
[C:539; E:212; G:237]

757   Hard, fixed and tender nodules may be felt on vaginal examination, particularly over the uterosacral ligaments. Fixed retroversion of the uterus can occur and ovarian enlargement may be detected. Laparoscopy is the most appropriate diagnostic tool and, as already stated, may reveal endometriosis in a number of patients with no physical signs.

758   As most patients are young and wish to obtain or retain reproductive capabilities, conservative management is favoured. Pregnancy frequently has a beneficial effect on the condition and hormonal therapy aims at inducing a pseudopregnancy in terms of the endometrium. Continuous use of a combined oral contraceptive pill may be effective but breakthrough bleeding and other side effects are common. Progestogenic agents such as high dose norethisterone are used and more recently a pituitary gonadotrophin antagonist (danazol) has been widely acclaimed. Unfortunately side effects are common. Surgery is indicated, particularly in cases of subfertility, for removal of pelvic adhesions. Isolated spots can be diathermised via the laparoscope. Bowel surgery may be necessary particularly in cases of obstruction. Radical surgery is only indicated in women who do not desire further pregnancies or in whom symptoms become unbearable. This should be carried out after hormonal therapy has been tried.
[C:544; E:215; H:628]

759   This is a very rare condition, probably not related to adenomyosis, in which the myometrium becomes invaded with stromal cells. It has been considered to be a low grade sarcoma. The growth may extend into the broad ligament and the cut surface of the tumour shows worm-like masses of tumour. Hysterectomy and bilateral salpingo-oophorectomy is the treatment of choice and radiotherapy may be of some use. The prognosis must be guarded.
[C:548; H:448]

N   Uterine displacements, prolapse and associated urinary problems

760   This entirely depends upon whether the uterus is mobile or not. Mobile retroversion is a normal finding in 20 per cent of women during the reproductive phase of life and is not, as previously believed, a cause of infertility, recurrent abortion, backache, urinary problems etc. However, fixed retroversion is a pathological condition caused by adhesions binding the uterous down or by pelvic tumours lying anterior to the uterus. Causes of the former include endometriosis and pelvic inflammatory disease.
[E:227; G:102; H:367; J:271]

761   Dyspareunia may occur with mobile retroversion when the ovaries lie between the body of the uterus and the posterior fornix of the vagina. It is often forgotten that ovaries are delicate organs and, like testicles, are painful when traumatised. Before any operation is carried out to correct retroversion, a Hodge pessary should be fitted. This will temporarily antevert the uterus and, if the symptoms are alleviated, then surgery is worthwhile. Pelvic pain is the hallmark of conditions such as endometriosis and pelvic inflammatory disease and the surgical correction of retroversion is part of the treatment of the causative disease.
[E:229; J:271]

762   This is a condition in which the vagina or uterus or both descend and may become apparent outside the introitus. Many patients believe that prolapse must involve the uterus but this is not the case, and many prolapses involve the vagina alone.
[C:631; E:229; G:91; J:253]

763   The name given to any type of vaginal wall prolapse is dependent upon the underlying structure that it carries with it. Therefore anterior wall prolapses are either urethroceles, cystoceles or cystourethroceles. Similarly, posterior wall prolapses are known as rectoceles and prolapses of the posterior fornix are known as enteroceles and contain small bowel.
[C:631; E:229; H:353]

764 In this instance, the uterus descends down the vagina and inevitably takes vagina with it. Three degrees are recognised. A first degree prolapse occurs when the cervix descends to the introitus, a second degree when it passes through the introitus and a third degree (or procidentia) when the entire uterus (and vagina) lie outside the introitus.

Prior to uterine descent, the axis of the uterus must come into line with that of the vagina and it thus acts like a piston in a cylinder. Elongation of the supravaginal cervix is a feature of uterine prolapse as is stretching and elongation of the supporting transverse cervical and uterosacral ligaments. The broad and round ligaments have virtually no role in supporting the uterus but they inevitably become stretched as the uterus descends.
[C:631; E:230; G:91; H:369; J:253]

765 Apart from congenital weaknesses (as in spina bifida) the most important causes are parturition and the menopause. Obesity, excessive straining and pelvic tumours are all contributory.
[C:631; E:230; G:96]

766 With a remarkable consistency, patients complain of 'something coming down' or of a bearing down sensation and also of a lump appearing at the introitus, especially when straining at stool. Backache, which worsens with standing during the day and is relieved by lying flat in bed, is very typical. Bleeding from an ulcerated cervix may occur in cases of procidentia, caused by friction of the cervix on underwear. Urinary symptoms are most common and are discussed in later questions.
[C:632; E:232; G:97; J:259]

767 In cases of anterior or posterior wall prolapse with no urinary symptoms, simple colporrhaphy is performed. The operation consists of removing a section of vaginal skin, plicating the underlying fascia and suturing the skin edges. If there is uterovaginal prolapse, then vaginal hysterectomy may be performed with or without additional colporrhaphy. In some cases, where apparent uterine descent is due to cervical hypertrophy, colporrhaphy is

combined with cervical amputation (the Manchester repair operation). In the very old and debilitated, where surgery is considered an unnecessary risk, a ring pessary can be fitted. This needs removing and replacing every 4 months and may lead to chronic ulceration of the vagina. With modern anaesthesia, particularly in association with regional block, operation is almost always possible.
[C:638; E:233; G:99; H:373; J:261]

768 The patient should be admitted to hospital and the prolapse reduced manually. The vagina is then packed with a gauze roll soaked in an oestrogen containing cream. This will allow the oedema to subside, the ulcer to heal and the oestrogen will help keratinisation of the vaginal epithelium. If the condition of the patient allows, surgery may be undertaken after about 2 weeks.

769 The patient may have stress incontinence, urge incontinence (unstable bladder), a neurological bladder (e.g. in cases of transection of the cord), or a vaginal fistula communicating with the urinary tract. Many patients have a combination of stress incontinence and an unstable bladder. Retention with overflow is uncommon.

770 A number of factors are at play. These will include the action of the levator ani muscles when there is sudden stress, the natural tone of the urethra, the length of the urethra, the shape of the proximal urethra (i.e. whether there is funnelling of the bladder neck or not), the length of urethra that is intra-abdominal (i.e. above the level of the levatores ani muscles) and the angle between the urethra and bladder.
[C:646; G:339]

771 Stress incontinence is a condition in which small quantities of urine are voided involuntarily when the intra-abdominal pressure is suddenly raised as in coughing, sneezing, running, laughing, jumping dancing etc. The patient, once aware that urine is being voided, is able to control the stream immediately.
[C:647; E:261; H:357; J:653]

772 Whether the operation is performed vaginally

or retropubically, all aim to achieve lengthening of the urethra. The urethrovesical angle will also be improved and by approximation of the levatores ani, tone will increase. That portion of the urethra lying above the levatores ani is said to be intra-abdominal. When there is sudden stress, the pressure exerted on the bladder is also exerted on this portion of urethra. The two forces negate each other and opening of the bladder neck (which shortens the effective length of the urethra) is prevented. Therefore operations designed to lengthen the urethra and return the proximal urethra to an intra-abdominal position should relieve stress incontinence.
[C:649]

773 The vaginal approach includes anterior colporrhaphy and is often the primary choice in patients with prolapse. The urethra is buttressed by interrupted sutures placed in the pubocervical fascia or pubococcygeus muscle. This has the effect of compressing the urethra, lengthening it and improving the urethrovesical angle. Retropubic repairs include colposuspension (probably the best), sling operations using fascia or inert materials and plicating of paraurethral tissue and suturing it to the back of the pubis (Marshall–Marchetti–Kranz procedure).
[C:651; G:342; H:360; J:663]

774 This is not a mechanical problem as exists in pure stress incontinence but one caused by inappropriate action of the detrusor muscle. On sudden bladder filling or rise in intra-abdominal pressure, the detrusor contracts and the intravesical pressure overcomes the intra-urethral pressure and urine is voided.
[C:650; E:260; H:360; J:651]

775 She will typically complain of urgency, frequency and nocturia. There may be pre- and post-micturition discomfort. There is often a past history of recurrent cystitis, and/or childhood enuresis. Incontinence may occur, even when sitting or lying.
[C:650; H:360; J:652]

776 Various drugs have been employed and fall

into three groups—the anticholinergics (eme-probrium bromide), sympathomimetics (or-ciprenaline) and antiprostaglandins (indo-methacin). Mixed results are reported. Frequency and nocturia are often improved but urgency less often.

Mechanical overstretching of the bladder can be performed under epidural anaesthesia but results are disappointing. Of greatest success has been bladder training, often in conjunction with anticholinergic drugs. Patients are confined to hospital and over a period of time (about 2 weeks or more) are encouraged to hold urine for longer and longer periods.
[C:650]

777 Cystometry and urethral flow rates are of greatest help. These tests are enhanced by video- or cine-radiography which demonstrates the bladder neck and degree of descent with straining. One of these tests should always be carried out if previous surgery has failed to improve incontinence.
[J:659]

778 This condition occurs partly as a result of lack of oestrogens. The patient has frequency, nocturia and dysuria. Examination reveals urethral stenosis, trabeculation of the bladder (evidence of outlet obstruction) and a pale featureless bladder base. Treatment is urethrotomy, oestrogen replacement therapy and bladder training.
[E:262]

O The climacteric and menopause

779 The menopause is the cessation of menstruation; the climacteric is a period of life, which includes the menopause, marking the waning of ovarian function and the change from an ovulatory to an anovulatory state.
[C:593; E:282]

780 The responsiveness of the ovaries to gonadotrophins decreases. This leads to a fall in oestrogen levels which, in turn, stimulates a rise in gonadotrophin secretion and an alteration in their ratio, with a large rise in FSH levels. The

ovarian follicles become more and more resistant to gonadotrophins until first ovulation ceases and then menstruation stops. Oestrogen production by the ovaries declines to almost nil but synthesis of oestrogen after the menopause does continue, mainly by peripheral conversion of androgenic precursors formed by the adrenal gland and ovaries. This conversion takes place in subcutaneous fat.
[C:594; E:283]

781 The breasts tend to decrease in size and become pendulous. The uterus atrophies, the body particularly so that the ratio in size of cervix to body reverses and becomes 2 : 1. The endometrium diminishes drastically and becomes quiescent after the menopause. The vaginal skin becomes thin and depleted of glycogen. The pH rises due to the loss of lactobacilli and the vagina is more prone to pathogenic infection. Atrophic changes also affect the urethra, the vulva and pelvic supporting tissues.
[C:603; E:283]

782 Probably no more than 25 per cent, although widespread publicity given to hormonal replacement therapy may have led a higher proportion of women to seek advice.
[H:797]

783 Apart from cessation of menstruation, they are hot flushes, night sweats and insomnia.

784 Mood changes, irrationality, loss of memory, depression, lassitude and inability to concentrate are commonly quoted but it is difficult to decide whether this is the result of hormone depletion or the social and cultural surroundings in which the patient may find herself. She may be left at home, the children having grown up and left, without any adequate training for work outside the house. Boredom and a sense of frustration lead to the so-called 'empty nest' syndrome and may cause the symptoms described above. Loss of libido can occur in some, perhaps as a result of dyspareunia. However, if a woman remains sexually active, shrinkage of the vagina is unlikely to occur.
[C:612; E:285; G:50; H:797]

785   There is now overwhelming evidence that oestrogens have an anticatabolic effect, preventing the loss of calcium. Bilateral oophorectomy in a premenopausal woman leads to an increase in blood and urinary levels of both calcium and phosphorous. Serum alkaline phosphatase levels rise and there is decreased bone absorption of calcium and phosphorous. This negative calcium balance can be reversed by administration of small quantities of oestrogens.
[C:604; H:804]

786   It is suggested that postmenopausal women may lose a protective factor present in reproductive life and it is probably oestrogen. Reproductive women have higher levels of high density lipoprotein (HDL) than men of the same age and lower levels of cholesterol and very low density lipoproteins (VLDL). After the menopause these sex differences tend to diminish.
[C:609; H:810]

787   Hormone replacement therapy is intended to give the minimum dose of hormone necessary to relieve symptoms.
[E:287]

788   In any woman with a normal reproductive tract (known by some illuminating convention as the unhysterectomised woman), treatment must be on a cyclical basis (i.e. 3 weeks out of every 4). In the latter 7–10 days a progestogen is added to the oestrogen being given. This will, of course, produce withdrawal bleeding in most women.
      In view of the possible impact on the breast of unopposed oestrogens, many practitioners would favour a similar regimen for patients without a uterus.
[C:616; H:801]

789   These are the physiological oestrogens such as oestradiol, and oestrone; the conjugated equine oestrogens mainly derived from pregnant mare's urine; the synthetic oestrogens such as ethinyloestradiol, mestranol and diethylstilboestrol.
[H:801]

790   In   patients   receiving   oestrogens   alone,

whether continuously or cyclically, abnormal endometrial hyperplasia has been noted. This must be considered to be a precursor of endometrial carcinoma. In a retrospective study in the USA, the incidence of endometrial carcinoma was considerably greater in women treated with unopposed oestrogen than in a matched untreated group.
[C:617; H:803]

791 Mild sedatives and anxiolytics are commonly used. Clonidine may help hot flushes and β-adrenergic blocking agents may control some cardiovascular problems, particularly palpitations.
[C:623]

P Fertility control

Subfertility

792 Assuming normal cohabitation and the absence of coital problems, the probability (calculated from life-tables) of a woman becoming pregnant after 12 months is 82 per cent (in USA 93 per cent) and after 24 months is 95 per cent. Therefore it is reasonable to assume that after 12 months, if conception has not occurred, subfertility should be suspected.

793 The volume of ejaculate varies from 0·5 ml to 5 ml. Sperm density should be between 20 and 180 million per ml. The motility, up to 4 hours after ejaculation, should exceed 50 per cent. The morphology of sperms is a subject upon which there is no close agreement but it is accepted that an abnormal count not exceeding 25 per cent is within the normal range. Other factors of slightly less importance are liquefaction of the specimen, pH and fructose content. If leucocytes are present, semen culture must be undertaken.
[C:551; E:108; H:704; J:589]

794 Azoospermia may be the result of either blockage of the ducts or testicular failure. Small testicular size and a raised FSH strongly suggest primary testicular failure and surgical exploration is not worthwhile.

Klinefelter's syndrome or testicular maldescent may lead to this. Despite popular mythology, mumps orchitis is uncommonly associated with azoospermia. If the FSH level is normal and the testes of normal size, surgical exploration may be helpful. If the vas is *not* patent, vasoepididymostomy may achieve an improvement in the semen analysis.
[H:705]

795 At least four analyses should be performed before making the diagnosis because of the wide variation in individual analyses. If the density remains low, physical examination of the patient may reveal a varicocele. However, ligation of a varicocele does not necessarily mean a return to normal fertility. Impressive results have been reported with drugs such as arginine, mesterolone, antioestrogens (clomiphene citrate and tamoxifen) and systemic gonadotrophins but double blind controlled trials have failed to demonstrate the success claimed for these drugs.
[C:536; H:706]

796 In cases where there is a reduced count or low mortility, artificial insemination of a portion of the ejaculate through the cervical canal may result in a pregnancy. General advice about the wearing of loose underclothing, the avoidance of extra hot baths, daily douching of the testicles in cold water etc., owe more to folklore than fact. In rare cases, where sperm auto-antibodies exist, high dose steroid therapy may help.

797 Investigation is concerned with abnormalities of the ovulatory mechanism; abnormalities of the reproductive tract and abnormalities of sperm transport.

798 The basal body temperature chart should show a biphasic response with an elevated temperature for the latter 14 days of the cycle. Plasma progesterone level on day −7 (i.e. 21st day of a normal length menstrual cycle) should be in excess of 30 nmol/l. Endometrial biopsy taken premenstrually should show secretory changes compatible with the stated day of the cycle. A midcycle urine assay of LH levels is

now available to indicate follicular rupture. Laparoscopy immediately after supposed ovulation should demonstrate follicular rupture (marked by a punctum on the corpus luteum).
[C:552; G:278; H:697]

799   A clinical thermometer must be used. The temperature is recorded sublingually every morning on awakening and before getting out of bed, eating, drinking or smoking. The record starts on the first day of menses and continues until the next period starts when a new chart is begun.
[C:553; E:114; G:280; H:699]

800   The temperature remains relatively constant and fairly low for the first 12–14 days. There is then a brief preovulatory dip followed by a steep rise in temperature of about one-half degree centigrade. This rise usually takes 1 or 2 days and is maintained for the 14 days of the luteal phase.

801   First, they are only a very rough guide to ovulation and must not be considered to be anything more. The patient may get very intolerant of daily temperature recording and if this is how she feels, they should be abandoned. It may, for some patients, place too great an emphasis on sexual activity only at ovulation time and lead to psychosexual problems.
[E:114]

802   Serum prolactin levels should always be assessed. Gonadotrophin levels may be useful as well as thyroid function tests. Assays of testosterone and oestrogen metabolites may be necessary but these depend largely upon the clinical picture.
[E:116]

803   This level of progesterone suggests a defect in ovulation. There are a number of ovulation inducing drugs available, the two most commonly used being clomiphene and tamoxifen. They are given for 5 days as early as possible in the cycle (usually days 2 to 6 inclusive). A small dose (50 mg per day in the

235

case of clomiphene) is usual to start and the response monitored with repeated plasma progesterone levels and daily basal body temperature recording.

804   There are few side effects but flushes and headaches do sometimes occur. The incidence of multiple pregnancy is about 5 per cent and, almost all cases are twin pregnancies. Ovarian enlargement is a rare but recognised complication and regular bimanual examination should be carried out on patients undergoing treatment.

805   Systemic treatment with human menopausal gonadotrophins (a mixture of FSH and LH) augmented with a preovulatory injection of human chorionic gonadotrophins (similar to LH) may be used occasionally. The success rate in selected patients with amenorrhoea is as much as 70 per cent but falls when patients with oligomenorrhoea and anovulatory regular cycles are treated. The treatment must be very carefully monitored because of the risks of hyperstimulation which include multiple pregnancy (up to 25 per cent of patients). It is only used in specialised centres.

806   This is a test of sperm viability in the cervical mucus. It must be carried out in the 2–3 days prior to ovulation. The patient is instructed to have intercourse 6–14 hours prior to the test and not wash, bathe or douche after intercourse. A sample of cervical mucus is then obtained and examined microscopically. A minimum of three or four motile and progressive sperms should be seen in each high power field examined.
[C:551]

807   It is plentiful and clear. It has elastic properties such that it can be stretched the length of the vagina. On microscopy, large squamous cells with pyknotic nuclei may be noted and there are usually no other cells present.
[E:110; J:597]

808   Small preovulatory doses of oestrogen (oestrone piperazine sulphate 3 mg or ethinyloestradiol $10\,\mu g$) can be given for 4 days. This may

236

have the added advantage of enhancing the midcycle surge of LH.
[C:557; E:110]

809   Either a much reduced sperm concentration or absence of sexual intercourse. Inadequate vaginal penetration may be the case in the very obese.

810   This suggests the presence of sperm anti-bodies. Transcervical artificial insemination of the partner's sperm may help. Barrier contraception for 6 months is said to reduce antibody levels and may occasionally help. The use of steroids either systemically or topically does not seem to be efficacious.
[H:710]

811   (a) Gas insufflation.
       (b) Hysterosalpingography.
       (c) Laparoscopy and dye insufflation.
       [C:553; E:111; H:714]

812   (a) Gas insufflation. At best, it may confirm patency of one tube. It is highly inaccurate, gives little useful information and may cause gas embolisation of uterine veins. It should be considered of historical interest only.
       (b) Hysterosalpingography. This demonstrates the cavity of the uterus well and both tubes may be visualised throughout their length. It is often very painful when performed without anaesthesia, tubal spasm may occur and up to 50 per cent give erroneous facts.
       (c) Laparoscopy. The tubes and ovaries can be inspected as can the whole pelvic cavity. Extratubal causes (e.g. adhesions, endometriosis) can be identified. Accurate assessment of the site of tubal blockage can be ascertained. The uterine cavity cannot be displayed. The procedure usually requires a general anaesthesia and there are the attendant risks of laparoscopy.

813   Acute infective causes include salpingitis and peritonitis from other causes. Previous abdominal and particularly pelvic surgery can lead to adhesion formation. Endometriosis

may be widespread and lead to tubal blockage. Occasionally the blockage is congenital.
[H:714]

814   This largely depends upon the site of the blockage and its cause. If the fimbrial ends are sealed as a result of previous peritonitis (e.g. from acute appendicitis) the prognosis is reasonably good. If tubal blockage is caused through endosalpingitis (i.e. an ascending infection) the prospect is usually poor. However, improved microscopic techniques have generally improved the overall outlook. Where the tubes are totally diseased or have been previously removed, *in vitro* (extracorporeal) fertilisation and embryo transfer may help a few patients.
[C:557; H:716]

Contraception

815   The Pearl Index. This is the failure rate in terms of pregnancy in 100 fertile women using a particular method for one year (13 cycles).
[C:505; G:316; J:610]

816   The combined oestrogen–progestogen pill is the most effective and widely used. It is taken cyclically (for 3 weeks out of every 4). The continuous progestogen-only pill may be used by patients in whom the combined pill is unsuitable. An intramuscular injection of progestogen in an oily base will provide contraception for up to 3 months but is only suitable in certain circumstances.
[C:511; E:123; G:318; H:835; J:620]

817   The patient should be warned that she may experience slight nausea, breast tenderness and an initial weight gain of a pound or two. The withdrawal bleeding at the end of the cycle is usually slighter and less painful than normal menses.
[C:513; H:839]

818   Depression, loss of libido, headaches, leg cramps, increased vaginal discharge, a tendency to monilial infections, chloasma are all

reported but it must be emphasised that millions of women take the 'Pill' without any trouble.

Major complications of the Pill are hypertension, venous thrombosis, cerebrovascular accidents, cholestatic jaundice. Post-pill amenorrhoea was once considered to be a side effect but it is now believed that such an entity exists in only a very few women. The Pill masks the amenorrhoea producing regular withdrawal bleeding and the condition is only apparent on stopping the pill. The pregnancy rate for previous pill users over a 2-year period is the same as that for women previously using barrier methods, although the rate in the first 3 months after stopping oral contraception is slightly lower.
[C:513; F:125; G:320; H:839; J:621]

819   A history of venous thrombosis, oestrogen dependent tumours, liver disease, severe diabetes mellitus, and severe hypertension are absolute contraindications. Patients who are over 35 years old are generally advised not to take the Pill but this particularly applies if they smoke. Migraine sufferers may find that their condition is made worse by the Pill. Varicose veins themselves are not a contraindication.
[C:512]

820   It inhibits ovulation by preventing the LH surge at midcycle, it acts on the cervical mucus to make it hostile to sperm, it alters the normal endometrial development making successful nidation unlikely and it possibly alters tubal motility.
[E:124; H:837]

821   This acts on the cervical mucus, making it hostile to sperm penetration, and renders the endometrium unsuitable for ovum implantation.
[C:512; G:319]

822   Menstrual control is poor and many patients experience breakthrough bleeding or delay in menstruation. Occasionally patients may develop amenorrhoea. In these, the tiny amount of progestogen present in this pill is sufficient to suppress pituitary activity and

ovulation is prevented. Although the patient worries because she fears she may be pregnant (i.e. because of the absence of bleeding) she is, in effect, less likely to get pregnant than those patients who menstruate regularly on this preparation.

823 For the combined pill, the failure rate is about 0·1 per 100 women-years. For the continuous pill it is about 2 per 100 women-years.
[E:130]

824 Ethinyloestradiol is the most popular oestrogen at doses varying between 20 and 50 μg. The most commonly used pills contain 30 μg. The progestogens vary and the most common are norgestrel, norethisterone (norethindrone), norethisterone acetate and lynoestrenol.
[C:511; E:129; H:837]

825 If she takes it within 12 hours of the time that she normally does, then there is no reduction in efficiency. However, if the time elapsed is greater than 12 hours, she should still take the pill but extra methods of contraception (e.g. the sheath) should be used until the start of withdrawal bleeding, or for 14 days whichever is the sooner.

826 The most common cause is failure of absorption through vomiting or diarrhoea. Certain drugs may interfere with the metabolism of the pill, such as the antiepileptics, making it less reliable. Very occasional reports suggest that certain antibiotics may also lessen its efficiency.
[C:513; G:322]

827 In the UK, medroxyprogesterone 150 mg may be given to a woman whose partner has had a vasectomy and is awaiting his sperm count to fall to zero. It may also be used in women who have been vaccinated against rubella. Its use in other parts of the world has been much more widespread as it does afford a very high degree of protection. The effects of very prolonged use are, as yet, not well documented.
[C:517; E:129; G:320]

828 The sheath or condom, the vaginal diaphragm, and the cervical cap are available. All must be

used in conjunction with a spermicidal (cream, foam, pessary or jelly). The failure rate is between 4 and 8 per 100 women-years.
[C:506; E:120; H:833; J:610]

829 These fall into three groups:
(a) the inert plastic devices such as Lippe's loop and the Saf-T-coil.
(b) the metal bearing devices such as the Copper 7 and Copper T. Some more recent devices incorporate both copper and silver.
(c) hormone containing devices. These devices contain pure progesterone which is released very slowly but initial problems have been experienced with a higher tubal pregnancy rate.
[C:507; E:130; G:322; H:834; J:614]

830 Menorrhagia, dysmenorrhoea, the presence or history of pelvic inflammatory disease, fibroids that distort the cavity of the uterus, congenital abnormalities of the uterus, pregnancy all contraindicate use of IUCDs. Many would consider that nulliparity is a relative contraindication. Considerable caution must be exercised if fitting a patient who has valvular heart disease.
[C:509; J:616]

831 The immediate problems are of cramp-like pain and syncopal attacks. The long term problems are dysmenorrhoea and menorrhagia. Both are less likely to occur with small devices. Infection is relatively uncommon but does occur and presents a considerable threat to future fertility (hence the contraindication in nulliparous patients). Expulsion of the device occurs in about 9 per cent of patients. Translocation of the device through the uterine wall is a risk and if the threads of the device cannot be found, it must be considered. The pregnancy rate is about 2 per 100 women-years. If pregnancy does occur the device should be removed as soon as possible if the threads are visible.
[C:510]

832 Gentle searching of the cervical canal with artery forceps may reveal their presence. Various devices for intrauterine exploration are

241

available and most rely on some form of hook. Suction curettage with a 4 mm soft catheter will often locate the thread. If all these procedures fail, anteroposterior pelvic X-ray (preferable with a sound in the uterus) will confirm its presence or absence. If the IUCD is outside the uterus then it must be removed. This is usually possible via the laparoscope. Ultrasound scanning is also a useful tool for IUCD location. [C:510]

833   They are smaller and therefore eaiser to insert. Menstrual problems are less frequent. The pregnancy rate is lower. However, they have to be changed every 2–3 years, expulsion is more common and perforation more likely. [C:509]

834   Most definitely not. There is no indication for removal of an inert device if there are no clinical problems. In this case it may be left *in situ* until 1 year after the cessation of menstruation.

835   The rhythm method relies upon abstaining from intercourse during the fertile days of the month. In general, for a woman with a regular 28-day cycle, this means between days 10 and 18 of the cycle. However, for greater efficiency, a basal body temperature chart should be kept, but this is of little use in the years prior to the cessation of menses because of the occurrence of anovulatory cycles. Studies in the changes of cervical mucus provide a relatively good guide to the ovulatory state. Whatever method is used, the failure rate is between 5 and 10 per 100 woman-years. [C:506; G:317; J:610]

836   It is not safe because spermatozoa may be released prior to ejaculation and the method depends upon the self-control of the man. It may lead to tension and anxiety, impotence and frigidity and menstrual disturbances. It is very widely practised and is probably the oldest form of contraception known. [E:120; H:832; J:610]

837   It is a safe, simple outpatient procedure with a very high success rate and very low morbidity.

It must only be carried out after very careful counselling of the man and with his informed consent. There is often pain and swelling for 48 hours but little other discomfort. Haematoma formation and sepsis are rare.

Some form of contraception must be used until sterility is achieved and this depends upon the number of ejaculations that take place after the operation. On average, most men have zero sperm counts after 3 months. Psychosexual problems are unusual and when they occur may represent inadequate pre-operative counselling.
[E:133; J:631]

838 These are numerous and depend upon the approach taken. Tubal interruption by the Pomeroy, Irving and Madlener operations may be carried out at laparotomy or minilaparotomy. Fimbriectomy is popular in some countries and may be carried out through the posterior fornix of the vagina. Laparoscopic methods are probably the most popular now and tubal occlusion can be achieved by electrocoagulation or by the application of spring-loaded (Hulka) clips or silastic (Falope) rings. The failure rate for laparoscopic sterilisation is higher than that by minilaparotomy but it can be carried out on a 'day-patient' basis and tubal destruction by clip or ring is small. Reversal of the operation is therefore a more successful procedure.
[C:518; G:326; J:629]

839 A careful menstrual history must be taken. If the patient has troublesome periods likely to necessitate future surgery, then sterilisation by hysterectomy may be more advisable. Previous pelvic surgery or infection may make the operation technically difficult particularly via the laparoscope. The age and parity of the patient must also be considered but the final decision must be between the patient and the surgeon.